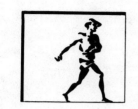

Dr. Heimlich's Home Guide to Emergency Medical Situations

by Henry J. Heimlich, M.D., with Lawrence Galton

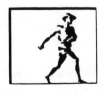

SIMON AND SCHUSTER • NEW YORK

Published by Simon and Schuster
A Division of Gulf & Western Corporation
Simon & Schuster Building
Rockefeller Center
1230 Avenue of the Americas
New York, New York 10020
SIMON AND SCHUSTER and colophon
are trademarks of Simon and Schuster

Designed by Irving Perkins
Manufactured in the United States of America

1   2   3   4   5   6   7   8   9   10

Library of Congress Cataloging in Publication Data

Heimlich, Henry J
    Dr. Heimlich's home guide to emergency medical situations.

    Includes index.
    1. Medical emergencies.   2. First aid in illness and injury.   I. Galton,
Lawrence, joint author.
    II. Title.
    RC86.7.H42   616'.025   79-21638

    ISBN 0-671-24947-9

Contents

Introduction: A Personal Word to the Reader

Behind this book lie a story and a concept. The concept has to do with the medical emergencies in your life—*all* the situations that really, and rightly, fall into the emergency category.

The story has to do with a tragic incident.

What has come to be known as the *Heimlich maneuver* was first described in June 1974, in a medical journal, *Emergency Medicine*. That same month, the simple huglike maneuver for saving the life of a person choking on food was successfully used by a lay person.

But at about the same time at a medical dinner meeting in Washington, D.C., a physician choked to death on a chunk of food as one hundred other physicians sat helplessly by, not realizing why their colleague had fallen unconscious and was dying.

The diagnosis of choking on food had been left so complex that even a large group of physicians failed to recognize the tragedy occurring in their midst.

Please bear with me for a moment about the story of the maneuver and how it relates to you.

The maneuver was developed after many laboratory studies. They showed that even in the midst of choking and inability to breathe, a substantial amount of air is left in the lungs. And they showed, too, that if you press your fist into a choking person's abdomen and thrust upward on the diaphragm, you compress the lungs and force the remaining air out through the windpipe—with such force that this air literally pops the obstruction out of the throat and mouth.

But if the maneuver were to be useful, recognition of choking had to be simplified so that the diagnosis could be made promptly by anyone—by a nearby diner in a restaurant, a family member at the dinner table at home, a mother whose child comes running because he is choking on a toy—for there are only four minutes to act. In four minutes life is lost.

It became possible, after analyzing what happens during choking, to establish a 1, 2, 3 order of events:

1. The person cannot breathe—*and cannot speak* (because his airway is blocked and no air can pass through the vocal cords).
2. He turns *blue* (because oxygen is not getting to body tissues).
3. He falls unconscious (because oxygen is not getting to his brain).

Then later, happily, the public contributed. As the maneuver became increasingly known, many people wrote. "Since the choking victim cannot speak," they suggested, "why not provide a signal he can use to indicate his condition to others." They suggested waving a finger, or hitting the top of the head with the flat of a hand, or throwing a plate against a wall.

It was with the help of a school for the deaf that I devised what is known now as the *Heimlich sign:* hand to neck. When a choking victim spreads a hand over the front of his neck, it says to anyone who has learned the signal (and millions now have): "Help me! I'm choking!" A potential rescuer then need only ask: "Are you choking?" And the victim can nod his head.

Both the 1, 2, 3 breakdown and sign as well as the maneuver have been much publicized through the media and through illustrated wall charts in public eating places and elsewhere.

The result has been a saving of more than 3,000 lives in the first four years.

Choking on food or another object is only one emergency situation. There are, of course, many more that involve life or death or serious disfigurement and disability—many of them long recognized to be situations requiring quick, knowledgeable treatment. You will find them in the pages that follow. You will also find more than one hundred other conditions beyond those ordinarily thought of as medical emergencies.

Yes, it is an emergency if you suffer a serious fall, a severe burn, break a limb, are badly bruised or cut. It is also an emergency if you suffer, or think you may be suffering, a heart attack; if you wake up in the middle of the night with a severe bellyache; if you get up in the morning with a stiff and painful neck; if suddenly a crop of hives covers your body. It can be an emergency if suddenly you develop severe itching, an outbreak of boils, a crop of painful canker sores, a headache that follows a seemingly minor head injury a few days before and refuses to vanish.

What this book tries to do is to break down such conditions to their basics: to make it easier for you to recognize what may be wrong; to guide you, whenever possible, to treating it successfully yourself; and to guide you, too, to recognizing when you really do need medical help—and how soon.

I think you may find, too, that in those situations where you do need medical or surgical help, you will benefit by a greater understanding of what goes into the physician's diagnosis and what goes into effective treatment.

I hope you will find that what was planned for this book— to make it complete, direct and practical, with a format to enable you to find what you need quickly*—is realized and valuable to you. This guide clearly is intended for use in emergencies when there is not time to obtain trained professional advice and help.

I think you will find the "Read This Now" pages that immediately follow especially valuable. And I urge you to read them first.

HENRY J. HEIMLICH, M.D.

* Entries are arranged alphabetically and cross-referenced where necessary. Also there is a comprehensive index at the back of the book.

Part One

Read
This
Now

Why Now

Almost certainly, there are many pages throughout this book to which you will be referring at some time in the future, and some you may have reason to consult now because they may serve an immediate need.

These next pages, however, are indeed special, and I hope very much that you will read them now and perhaps come back to review them at regular intervals.

They are important because they contain information you should know about in advance of emergency—facts, insights, procedures that can help you to act promptly, knowingly, effectively.

They are important, too, because they can help you in some situations to avoid well-meant but misguided, outdated advice and directions from other sources, including some you may, understandably enough, believe to be authentic.

And they are important, some in particular, for attitude of mind.

"Look at the Bleeding" is very much concerned with attitude. I think you will agree that it will be an attitude you will want to transmit to your children to serve them throughout their lives, and enable them to react to emergency situations and illness calmly, with understanding and without panic.

The section on POISONING can help you avoid mistakes— some of them potentially disastrous—that might not be your fault but rather due to outdated first aid labels, now known to be mistaken but still carried on many dangerous household products.

Your understanding of the section on SHOCK—on how to recognize as well as combat it—can make a life and death difference in many accidents and other medical emergency situations. Shock can be a needless killer.

The two sections on ABDOMINAL PAIN and CHEST PAIN will give you insights into their many possible causes and help you determine what is going on and what to do when either of these very common symptoms occurs.

CHOKING . . . AND THE HEIMLICH MANEUVER—here, too, it is essential to know in advance how to recognize the former

21

and how to apply the latter without even a few minutes' delay.

Similarly, the CPR (cardiopulmonary resuscitation) section belongs here because there is little time for you to first read about it when a life is at stake.

The section on BURNS prepares you to quickly size up the seriousness of a burn and, accordingly, what to do promptly for it.

SAVE THAT ACCIDENTALLY AMPUTATED BODY PART belongs here because no longer need the accidental amputation of a part of the body—finger, arm, leg, nose, ear—invariably mean permanent loss if you know a few basic procedures that you can follow that will allow physicians and surgeons to later use new reconnecting, reimplanting, and grafting techniques.

Perhaps at first blush the COUGHING section may seem out of place. Yet coughing is often misunderstood and mistreated. You will find it rewarding to know that there are times when you should not only *not* suppress but instead *encourage* it— and *HOW* to do that.

I have included here, too, suggestions on how to stock emergency kits—for your home, for your car, for usual travel, and for travel that may take you beyond medical aid.

"Look at the Bleeding!"

How we react—or how our parents react—when we first cut or injure ourselves and become aware of bleeding can affect our response to injuries and illnesses throughout our lives.

Do consider:

When a child comes running to a parent with a small amount of blood trickling through the skin—or, for that matter, a large amount—if the parent becomes alarmed and panicky, the tension will be transmitted immediately to the child who, for the rest of his or her life, is likely to react with the same alarm and panic at the sight of blood and in the face of other injury or illness.

If parent or child becomes sufficiently upset to faint, the situation is further worsened.

Yet a fairly substantial amount of blood can be lost—in an adult as much as a pint, in a child a little less—with little or no serious effect.

Should anyone in your family suffer an injury that leads to bleeding, simply hold the arm or leg or whatever other part of the body is bleeding, and say quietly: "Well, look at the blood; isn't that great! It washes out the wound so the germs which got in when you cut yourself will not stay in there."

Say to the child: "Do look. It's really a wonderful process. And now that it has done its work, we'll soon stop it."

When that child grows up, he will know how to react calmly and constructively to emergencies and, as well, to disease.

The first thing to do with any such cut or bruise is to wash it with clear, cold water and advise the child that this may cause a little burning sensation. Explain that the reason for the burning sensation is that the place where the skin is cut or broken has left some nerves exposed—but don't worry; they will heal.

If possible, wash the area surrounding the wound with soap and water. Do not be concerned if, as you rinse the soap off the surrounding area of skin, a little of the soap-containing rinse water washes into the wound; it further cleanses it.

For a cut, apply a sterile bandage and apply a little pressure until the bleeding stops. Usually, with small amounts of bleeding, clotting will occur within three minutes, ending the bleeding.

For a raw wound, don't use dry gauze because it will stick, and when you pull it off later it will take with it the clotted blood and allow bleeding to start again. Instead, use sterile petrolatum (Vaseline) gauze, or apply a sterile ointment and then cover with gauze. Also available are nonadherent bandages.

If the cut is deep and gapes open, you may do as well as your doctor does when he sutures or stitches if you follow this procedure:

After the wound has been cleaned and the skin is dry, apply one adhesive end of a small sterile Band-Aid, or equivalent, on one side near the cut. With your other hand, apply just enough pressure to hold the edges of the wound together so they just touch, taking care not to pinch them together too tightly nor touch the wound itself with your fingers. Then lay down the other adhesive end on the opposite side of the cut.

If you do this in such a way that the edges of the skin come together nicely, you may well achieve the equivalent of a professional plastic surgery repair. *Note:* Only close the edges of a fresh clean wound; to do this with an old or dirty wound will enclose the contamination and result in infection.

If the cut is on the face or another visible area, to be certain you have done the right thing you should see a physician. If necessary, he can insert small sutures in a way to avoid scarring.

When you proceed thus, in a calm and certain way, you will endow your child with a sense of security not only about the immediate accident but also for the sight of blood, for any injury, and for illness in the future. If, for example, the child should be involved in an auto accident in the future, it will be possible for him or her to calmly assess the injuries, personal and of others, avoiding the problems caused by crying and fainting.

This, of course, does not mean that you should have your children make light of accidents. They should become aware of hazards and be taught to avoid them.

But realistically, accidents are not always avoidable, nor are illnesses, and the confidence engendered by this "Look at the bleeding" approach will serve your children, and quite likely yourself, well. If your reaction to an emergency—even losing your auto keys—is one of panic, think back on your own life. How did you and your parents react at the time of your first injury? Make up your mind to calmly evaluate the situation and react productively when next faced with an unusual, acute problem.

Poisonings

Each year in the United States, more than a million cases of poisoning (85 percent of them among children) occur, leading to sickness and suffering for many thousands and death for several hundred.

And please note well: *Often matters can be made worse by following outdated, inaccurate first aid labels* on many potentially poisonous household products—*and even by following outdated and erroneous information in some widely used first aid manuals.*

Although much information about poisonings and how best to treat them has been obtained recently, the first aid labeling on many products has not been changed for years.

Note These Matters of Concern:

• The labeling on many alkaline household drain cleaners, oven cleaners, and products that contain lye prescribes, in case of accidental swallowing, use of vinegar or citrus fruit juice to provide a neutralizing effect. But the reaction of these natural acids with the alkali may increase gastrointestinal burning.

• Often, the final instruction is to follow the vinegar or juice with butter or a cooking oil, which is supposed to be soothing. But it is also a coating and concealer—and wrong since it interferes with the physician's ability to determine the extent of damage and what further treatment is essential.

• In case of poisoning with an acid-containing or acid-releasing product, even some medical texts still recommend use of sodium bicarbonate. But that carries the risk of blowing out the stomach.

• For people who swallow alcohol-based products such as antifreeze, there is a decade-old instruction to induce vomiting with a tablespoon of salt in a glass of water. But the Consumer Product Safety Commission has recently reported that *this could cause fatal salt poisoning*—and that it is not safe to use salt solutions to induce vomiting for any accidental ingestion.

• Should vomiting be induced after swallowing a product such as glue, paint, fondue fuel, or furniture polish containing a petroleum distillate? Labels differ. They probably should caution against inducing vomiting, but it is more essential to take another step: call a poison control center. Under some circumstances, if a large amount has been swallowed or the product also contains a dangerous additive, vomiting may be needed. But if done at home, vomiting of a petroleum distillate may cause some of it to be sucked into the lungs. In a hospital emergency room, precautions can be taken and vomiting or washing out of the stomach can be done safely.

What You Should Properly Do About Poisonings

First, consider it absolutely essential to be prepared—just by having two things always on hand—so you can be certain you are helping, not hurting:

1. An ounce bottle of syrup of ipecac, which your druggist can sell without prescription.
2. The phone number of the nearest poison control center. There are now some 600 centers across the country. You may find the number of the nearest in the front section of your telephone directory. If not, ask your physician.

A safe first aid procedure is to give one or two glasses of water to dilute the poison. Then, immediately call the poison control center—or a physician, hospital, or rescue unit. Be prepared to report as much as you can about what was swallowed: name of product, maker, contents if they are listed on the container. And, very important, how much was swallowed.

You may then be instructed, depending upon the nature of the poison, to induce vomiting.

To make a patient vomit, give one tablespoonful (½ ounce) of syrup of ipecac for a child a year of age or older, plus at least one cup of water. If no vomiting occurs in 20 minutes, repeat once only. Keep the patient walking, and if no vomiting has occurred within 10 minutes after the second dose of ipecac, try to induce vomiting by tickling the back of the throat. In the case of a child, when vomiting does occur, place in a "spanking position" with head lower than hips to avoid inhalation of vomitus.

If syrup of ipecac is not available, try to induce vomiting by tickling the back of the throat with a spoon handle or other blunt object after giving water. But don't waste time waiting for vomiting if it is delayed. Take the victim promptly to a hospital emergency room or physician, bringing along the poison's container with intact label. If the poison is not known, the examining physician will make judgments based on other clues.

Please note well: You will not be wasting time getting through to a poison control center for instructions. The centers carefully collect information about the contents of various products from manufacturers and, with this knowledge, are in a position to advise you on exactly what has to be done—at home or otherwise—in a specific case of poisoning. *Always, specific treatment is better than general treatment.*

If an eye is affected: Immediately wash the eye gently, using plenty of water (or milk in an emergency) for at least 15 minutes, with the eyelid held open. Call a poison control center, doctor, hospital or rescue unit and get the victim to a medical facility promptly.

If the skin is affected: Wash off immediately with a large amount of water. Use soap if available. Remove any contaminated clothing. And call for help.

If a poison has been inhaled: Get any victim who has inhaled such things as fuel gas, auto exhaust, dense smoke from a fire, or fumes from poisonous chemicals into fresh air. Loosen clothing. If breathing has stopped, start artificial respiration (p. 49) immediately. Don't stop until breathing starts or help arrives. And while doing this, have someone else call for help.

The Best Way to Prevent Poisoning at Home

Keep these facts in mind:

- Most poisonings involve children up to 3 years of age.
- The unpleasant taste of a potential poison is *not* a deterrent to a child.
- The most dangerous time is the hour before the evening meal—a time that one poison control center physician calls the "arsenic hour"—the time when a child is hungry. At this particular time, it may be a good idea to place cookies on the table for a child to grab.

Currently, medicines make up 50 percent of poison control center calls. At the top of the list: aspirin, tranquilizers, sedatives, sleeping pills, vitamins. Cleaning agents account for about 20 percent; insecticides, about 10 percent; petroleum distillates (gasoline, turpentine, lighter fluid, etc.) about 7 percent; the rest includes plants and cosmetics.

Keep all such items, all inedibles, in their original containers. (A common cause of poisoning is transfer of poisonous liquid to soft drink bottles.) And keep such items out of sight and out of a child's reach, with all medicines locked away.

Teach children never to take medicine unless given by an adult.

Shock

Medical shock—which has nothing to do with electrical shock—is a potentially grave emergency. It can cause death from injuries and illnesses that in themselves would not be fatal.

It is important for you to have some advance knowledge of what shock is, when it may occur, how to recognize it, and what to do for it.

WHAT IT IS: Shock is a depressed body state caused by upset of the mechanisms that keep blood circulating properly to all parts of the body. Because of the failure in circulation, the brain, heart, and other vital organs are deprived of adequate blood.

WHEN IT OCCURS: It may follow severe injury, severe burns, infection, pain, bleeding, stroke, heart attack, heat exhaustion, food or chemical poisoning, broken bones, exposure.

WHAT TO LOOK FOR: Paling of the face.

Cold, clammy skin with drops of sweat on forehead and palms of hands.

Restlessness, confusion, apprehension, trembling, nervousness or unconsciousness.

Pulse weak, small, rapid—referred to as "thready."

Nausea or vomiting.

Increased breathing rate, usually over 20 breaths a minute; breathing may also be irregular and with some deep sighing.

Sharp fall in blood pressure.

WHAT TO DO: Keep the victim lying down (if possible with head lower than the rest of the body) to encourage blood flow to the brain. A person with a *head injury* may be kept flat or propped up, but the *head* should *not* be lower than the rest of the body; otherwise swelling of the brain may occur.

Raise the legs 8 to 12 inches, supporting them on blankets or anything else handy, if there are no broken bones. This enables blood in the legs to reach the heart and major circulation. If there is increased breathing difficulty or pain when the legs are raised, lower them again.

If there is any bleeding, stop it if possible (see BLEEDING).

Cover the victim only enough to prevent loss of body heat if the weather is cold or damp. Don't overheat.

Check on the airway. If there is mucus or vomitus, remove it. A victim who is unconscious should be placed on his side to aid drainage of fluids out of the mouth and help avoid airway blockage by vomitus. If there is no risk of such blockage and the victim is having difficulty breathing, place him on his back, with head and shoulders raised on a blanket.

Fluids by mouth have value in shock but should be administered only under certain conditions: if medical help will not be available for an hour or more; if the victim is not vomiting or likely to vomit, and is not unconscious. Fluid given to an unconscious or semiconscious person may flow into the lungs, worsening the condition. Nor should fluid be administered if the victim appears to have a brain or abdominal injury.

The fluid should be water, neither hot nor cold—best of all, water containing one level teaspoonful of table salt and one-half level teaspoonful of baking soda to a quart. For an adult, give about half a glass every 15 minutes; for a child under 12, a quarter glass; for an infant, an eighth of a glass or one ounce. Stop fluid administration if the victim vomits or becomes nauseated.

A physician overcomes shock by giving intravenous fluids, administering blood if needed, and treating the primary condition that caused the shock.

Anaphylactic Shock

This is a grave emergency condition—a catastrophic, allergic, whole-body reaction that occurs in a previously sensitized person when he or she is again exposed to the same sensitizing material. The material may be an otherwise valuable drug such as penicillin, a serum, an anesthetic, or a sting from a honeybee, wasp, yellow jacket, or hornet.

THESE ARE THE INDICATIONS: Typically, within 1 to 15 minutes after exposure to a sensitizing material, a sense of uneasiness, agitation, flushing; giant hives all over the skin; swelling over the entire body; difficulty in breathing; coughing; sneezing; itching; nausea and vomiting (less common).

Then, within another minute or two, signs of shock may develop: paling of the face; cold, clammy skin; sweat on the forehead and palms; weak, rapid, small pulse.

Subsequently, the victim may convulse, become incontinent, unresponsive, and die. Someone in anaphylactic shock can be dead in minutes.

WHAT TO DO: Immediate treatment with epinephrine (Adrenalin) by injection under the skin is imperative.

Any person who has displayed sensitivity to a drug, serum, or anesthetic should always make that fact known to a treating physician and would do well to carry some indication of the fact—a card, bracelet, etc.

Anyone known to be sensitive to insect stings should always carry a sting kit when likely to be exposed. The kit, which must be prescribed by a physician, contains epinephrine, hypodermic needle, a strong antihistamine.

If a sting kit is available, 0.3 to 0.5 milliliters of 1:1,000 aqueous epinephrine should be injected under the skin (following directions in the kit), without loss of time—if possible, at the very first indication of anaphylactic reaction. A second injection may be needed for a severe reaction. And the victim should be taken to physician, emergency room, or other medical facility as quickly as possible.

If no kit is available, then during the trip to a medical facility, spread of the insect venom should be slowed by continuous ice or cold compresses applied to the site and by use of a

Chest Pain

This section, like that on abdominal pain, is an important one to be familiar with in advance of the occasion.

Almost the first thought that leaps into the mind of anyone experiencing chest pain is that the heart may be involved. It may be, of course; real heart disease is a vast enough problem. But according to some estimates as many as 20 million Americans, most of them men and many of them young, are bearing needless burdens of concern and limitation of activity because, although they may have experienced some of the symptoms, notably chest pain, they do not have anything wrong with their heart.

We will consider the chest pains of heart disease and their distinguishing features and also chest pains that have nothing to do with the heart and what distinguishes them.

Angina: the Pain of Coronary Heart Disease

The chest pain that may accompany disease of the coronary arteries which nourish the heart muscle (called coronary heart disease or CHD) is known as *angina pectoris*—"angina" standing for suffocating or choking pain and "pectoris" referring to the chest.

The situation that leads to anginal chest pain is somewhat analogous to what happens when the fuel line of a car becomes corroded inside, its inner wall thickening with rust deposits so there is less room for fuel to flow from the gas tank through the line to the engine. Enough fuel may get through at slow or moderate speed on a level road. But when there's a hill to climb or the driver accelerates, the motor sputters for lack of adequate fuel flow.

So may the heart sputter, causing anginal chest pain, under some circumstances when coronary heart disease is present, for in this disease the inner walls of the coronary arteries are encrusted to some degree with fatty deposits.

Angina is not like a heart attack, in which blood flow to an area of heart muscle is suddenly blocked off completely or

tourniquet above the sting. The tourniquet should be at least two inches wide. If a commercial tourniquet is not available, use a triangular bandage, towel, or handkerchief folded several times. Wrap snugly—not so tight, however, that the pulse cannot be felt. Loosen briefly every four minutes. In case of a bee sting, remove and discard the stinger and venom sac.

Abdominal Pain

What do you do if you suddenly develop a bellyache, perhaps wake up with it in the middle of the night? By studying this section before you have a problem, you will be familiar with possible causes and how to check on them and narrow in on the probable cause and what to do.

First, take a short medical history; ask the questions your doctor would ask if you were to call him. Look back a little: Did you eat a heavy meal or sizable snack just before going to bed, or were you at a party where you did more than your usual amount of eating and drinking?

If it's a youngster who has the pain, did he, say, go to a movie and gobble three boxes of popcorn and a chocolate bar and drink a lot of soda pop?

More often than not, sudden abdominal pain is likely to be from something you ate. If the pain is not extreme or localized to any one region but extends throughout much of the abdomen, you can try an antacid preparation or a glass of milk. Did you have a normal bowel movement in the past 48 hours? If not, use a suppository to induce one. Retention of stool is a common cause of abdominal pain.

Is the pain diminishing? If so, you are probably on your way to recovery; give it a little more time.

Whether it occurs at night or at other times, abdominal pain can have varied causes, some minor, some not to be taken lightly. And you can often determine what is likely to be the problem by considering where in the abdomen the pain is located, its nature, and any other symptoms that accompany it:

• When the pain is in the upper abdomen and accompanied

by other symptoms that may include nausea, heartburn, flatulence, belching, feelings of fullness and stomach distention, all developing during or after a meal, the problem can be indigestion. (See INDIGESTION.)

• When the pain occurs first in the area around the navel (belly button), accompanied or preceded by nausea or a feeling of "upset stomach," and then the pain *shifts* to the right lower quadrant or quarter of the abdomen, the problem can be appendicitis. (See APPENDICITIS.)

• If you have had an abdominal operation in the past, a possible cause of abdominal pain is formation of adhesions leading to intestinal obstruction. Such obstruction may sometimes occur from other causes. Symptoms depend upon whether the obstruction is in the small or large intestine and whether it is complete or partial:

—Severe, cramplike pain around the navel area that may come and go, vomiting that is recurrent and eventually becomes fecal, abdominal distention, and inability to pass gas or stool can indicate complete obstruction of the small intestine. With partial obstruction, symptoms are similar but less severe, and diarrhea may follow cramps.

—Pain lower in the abdomen, less severe, with abdominal distention, and with vomiting developing later may indicate obstruction of the colon or large bowel. If obstruction is complete, constipation is absolute and gas cannot be passed at all. With partial obstruction, bowel action may be irregular, with passage of frequent small stools. (See INTESTINAL OBSTRUCTION.)

• If you know you have a hernia—or if you discover a lump in the groin or in the navel—be sure to see the section on HERNIA.

• If your pain is in the right upper quadrant of the abdomen and it is preceded or accompanied by abdominal distention and by nausea with or without vomiting, the gallbladder may be involved. (See GALLBLADDER DISEASE.)

• In a woman, pain in the right or left lower abdomen, sudden and severe, and often accompanied by nausea and vomit-

---

ing, may be due to a twisted ovarian cyst. (CYSTS.)

• A severe pain that starts in the lower abdor ually extends upward to the right upper quadra of the abdomen, increasing in severity without r abdomen becoming tight and rigid as a board peritonitis, possibly due to a perforated ulcer. (S TIS.)

• When abdominal pain (which may be eith knifelike or deep and dull) is relieved by pass stool, and when such episodes are frequent and by any or many other symptoms such as diarrhe alternating with constipation, nausea, heartburi the problem could be irritable colon. (See COLON

• When severe pain is in the upper abdomer the area about the stomach, extending to the ba and is relieved when you sit up, it could be acute (See PANCREATITIS, ACUTE.)

• Sudden abdominal pain or cramps accompan many other symptoms such as nausea, vomitir gling" in the intestines, diarrhea, sometimes hea muscle aches, and prostration can indicate ga which can result from "intestinal grippe" or " virus, food poisoning, or gastrointestinal allerg TROENTERITIS, ACUTE; also ALLERGIES.)

WHAT TO DO: Consider calmly what the possil view of the symptoms.

If the problem lies with something you ate anc tions noted earlier help, fine.

If you can be certain that another nonseriou applies and it is of transient nature and will cure Otherwise:

1. Eat nothing.
2. Limit your fluid intake to small sips of water
3. Assume any position you find most comfortal
4. Do *not* take a laxative or enema.
5. Call your physician after noting as much as y the pain and its nature, other symptoms, yo ture, and what you think may be possible cau

severely restricted, damaging that nourishment-deprived area. Angina represents protest by, but not damage to, the heart muscle.

Angina usually appears, as may a heart attack, during exertion—running for a bus, climbing stairs, playing tennis, shoveling snow. The exertion requires increased work of the heart, which a well-nourished organ takes in stride. But the increased effort, which calls for increased nourishment, is difficult for the heart when the coronary arteries can't let through more blood.

Angina, as a rule, is felt as a constrictive sensation in the middle of the chest which often radiates, or shoots out, to the left arm and fingertips. But there are variations: occasionally, instead of in the chest, pain appears between the shoulder blades, in the left arm or shoulder, left hand or wrist, in the pit of the abdomen, in the jaws and teeth, or even in parts of the right arm.

Anginal chest pain has other characteristics. Usually, it is frightening as well as painful, triggering a sense of foreboding and compelling the victim to stop whatever he is doing.

Moreover, an attack is usually brief, over in a few minutes. It responds quickly to rest and, as well, to a nitroglycerin tablet. If chest pain persists for more than 15 minutes, it is not likely to be angina. You can be reassured that no heart attack is involved if the pain disappears quickly, but diagnosis by a physician is still warranted.

Heart Attack Chest Pain

The chest pain that is the hallmark of a heart attack can range from a slight feeling of pressure to a sensation that the chest is being crushed in a vise.

If an angina victim suffers a heart attack and at first assumes he is having just another angina attack, he should soon realize otherwise. This time, rest does no good, nor does nitroglycerin. Typically, the pain persists for hours and does not subside until a narcotic such as meperidine (Demerol) is administered.

Almost always with the chest pain there is grave anxiety, a

feeling that death is near. Commonly, the face turns ashen gray and a cold sweat appears. Often, retching, belching of gas, and vomiting develop and sometimes may make a victim think he is having a stomach upset. Shortness of breath is common. Sometimes, there may be palpitation—a sensation that the heart is beating abnormally fast and hard.

Some helps in distinguishing the chest pain of a heart attack from angina and from chest pains unrelated to the heart: It is less likely to be a heart attack if chest pain is below the nipple and to the left; if the pain is localized completely to the left; if the pain is sharp rather than a dull pressure or squeezing sensation; if the pain comes and goes; if the pain lessens when you lie down. If the pain persists for only one to five minutes, it is probably angina, not a heart attack.

What to Do for Angina

If you begin to experience what appear to be anginal chest pain attacks, based on the characteristics previously described, by all means see a physician for thorough examination and treatment.

Angina need not make an invalid of you nor seriously limit your activities. There are medications your physician can prescribe—nitroglycerin and others—which can be used safely and effectively not only to relieve angina but also to prevent recurrences. Other measures can help, including perhaps graduated exercise and change in diet and some practical changes in life-style.

What to Do for a Heart Attack

If you know—or even just suspect—you are having a heart attack, act promptly. The first hours and even minutes can sometimes be critical.

Ask someone to take you to the nearest hospital or call the rescue squad. And once you reach the emergency room, immediately tell personnel there that you may be having a heart attack and insist on being taken to the coronary care unit.

tourniquet above the sting. The tourniquet should be at least two inches wide. If a commercial tourniquet is not available, use a triangular bandage, towel, or handkerchief folded several times. Wrap snugly—not so tight, however, that the pulse cannot be felt. Loosen briefly every four minutes. In case of a bee sting, remove and discard the stinger and venom sac.

Abdominal Pain

What do you do if you suddenly develop a bellyache, perhaps wake up with it in the middle of the night? By studying this section before you have a problem, you will be familiar with possible causes and how to check on them and narrow in on the probable cause and what to do.

First, take a short medical history; ask the questions your doctor would ask if you were to call him. Look back a little: Did you eat a heavy meal or sizable snack just before going to bed, or were you at a party where you did more than your usual amount of eating and drinking?

If it's a youngster who has the pain, did he, say, go to a movie and gobble three boxes of popcorn and a chocolate bar and drink a lot of soda pop?

More often than not, sudden abdominal pain is likely to be from something you ate. If the pain is not extreme or localized to any one region but extends throughout much of the abdomen, you can try an antacid preparation or a glass of milk. Did you have a normal bowel movement in the past 48 hours? If not, use a suppository to induce one. Retention of stool is a common cause of abdominal pain.

Is the pain diminishing? If so, you are probably on your way to recovery; give it a little more time.

Whether it occurs at night or at other times, abdominal pain can have varied causes, some minor, some not to be taken lightly. And you can often determine what is likely to be the problem by considering where in the abdomen the pain is located, its nature, and any other symptoms that accompany it:

• When the pain is in the upper abdomen and accompanied

by other symptoms that may include nausea, heartburn, flatulence, belching, feelings of fullness and stomach distention, all developing during or after a meal, the problem can be indigestion. (See INDIGESTION.)

• When the pain occurs first in the area around the navel (belly button), accompanied or preceded by nausea or a feeling of "upset stomach," and then the pain *shifts* to the right lower quadrant or quarter of the abdomen, the problem can be appendicitis. (See APPENDICITIS.)

• If you have had an abdominal operation in the past, a possible cause of abdominal pain is formation of adhesions leading to intestinal obstruction. Such obstruction may sometimes occur from other causes. Symptoms depend upon whether the obstruction is in the small or large intestine and whether it is complete or partial:

—Severe, cramplike pain around the navel area that may come and go, vomiting that is recurrent and eventually becomes fecal, abdominal distention, and inability to pass gas or stool can indicate complete obstruction of the small intestine. With partial obstruction, symptoms are similar but less severe, and diarrhea may follow cramps.

—Pain lower in the abdomen, less severe, with abdominal distention, and with vomiting developing later may indicate obstruction of the colon or large bowel. If obstruction is complete, constipation is absolute and gas cannot be passed at all. With partial obstruction, bowel action may be irregular, with passage of frequent small stools. (See INTESTINAL OBSTRUCTION.)

• If you know you have a hernia—or if you discover a lump in the groin or in the navel—be sure to see the section on HERNIA.

• If your pain is in the right upper quadrant of the abdomen and it is preceded or accompanied by abdominal distention and by nausea with or without vomiting, the gallbladder may be involved. (See GALLBLADDER DISEASE.)

• In a woman, pain in the right or left lower abdomen, sudden and severe, and often accompanied by nausea and vomiting, may be due to a twisted ovarian cyst. (See OVARIAN CYSTS.)

• A severe pain that starts in the lower abdomen and gradually extends upward to the right upper quadrant and middle of the abdomen, increasing in severity without relief, with the abdomen becoming tight and rigid as a board, can indicate peritonitis, possibly due to a perforated ulcer. (See PERITONITIS.)

• When abdominal pain (which may be either sharp and knifelike or deep and dull) is relieved by passage of gas or stool, and when such episodes are frequent and accompanied by any or many other symptoms such as diarrhea or diarrhea alternating with constipation, nausea, heartburn, headaches, the problem could be irritable colon. (See COLON, IRRITABLE.)

• When severe pain is in the upper abdomen, sharpest in the area about the stomach, extending to the back and chest, and is relieved when you sit up, it could be acute pancreatitis. (See PANCREATITIS, ACUTE.)

• Sudden abdominal pain or cramps accompanied by any or many other symptoms such as nausea, vomiting, gas "gurgling" in the intestines, diarrhea, sometimes headache, fever, muscle aches, and prostration can indicate gastroenteritis, which can result from "intestinal grippe" or "stomach flu" virus, food poisoning, or gastrointestinal allergy. (See GASTROENTERITIS, ACUTE; also ALLERGIES.)

WHAT TO DO: Consider calmly what the possibilities are in view of the symptoms.

If the problem lies with something you ate and the suggestions noted earlier help, fine.

If you can be certain that another nonserious possibility applies and it is of transient nature and will cure itself, fine. Otherwise:

1. Eat nothing.
2. Limit your fluid intake to small sips of water or ice chips.
3. Assume any position you find most comfortable.
4. Do *not* take a laxative or enema.
5. Call your physician after noting as much as you can about the pain and its nature, other symptoms, your temperature, and what you think may be possible causes.

Chest Pain

This section, like that on abdominal pain, is an important one to be familiar with in advance of the occasion.

Almost the first thought that leaps into the mind of anyone experiencing chest pain is that the heart may be involved. It may be, of course; real heart disease is a vast enough problem. But according to some estimates as many as 20 million Americans, most of them men and many of them young, are bearing needless burdens of concern and limitation of activity because, although they may have experienced some of the symptoms, notably chest pain, they do not have anything wrong with their heart.

We will consider the chest pains of heart disease and their distinguishing features and also chest pains that have nothing to do with the heart and what distinguishes them.

Angina: the Pain of Coronary Heart Disease

The chest pain that may accompany disease of the coronary arteries which nourish the heart muscle (called coronary heart disease or CHD) is known as *angina pectoris*—"angina" standing for suffocating or choking pain and "pectoris" referring to the chest.

The situation that leads to anginal chest pain is somewhat analogous to what happens when the fuel line of a car becomes corroded inside, its inner wall thickening with rust deposits so there is less room for fuel to flow from the gas tank through the line to the engine. Enough fuel may get through at slow or moderate speed on a level road. But when there's a hill to climb or the driver accelerates, the motor sputters for lack of adequate fuel flow.

So may the heart sputter, causing anginal chest pain, under some circumstances when coronary heart disease is present, for in this disease the inner walls of the coronary arteries are encrusted to some degree with fatty deposits.

Angina is not like a heart attack, in which blood flow to an area of heart muscle is suddenly blocked off completely or severely restricted, damaging that nourishment-deprived area. Angina represents protest by, but not damage to, the heart muscle.

Angina usually appears, as may a heart attack, during exertion—running for a bus, climbing stairs, playing tennis, shoveling snow. The exertion requires increased work of the heart, which a well-nourished organ takes in stride. But the increased effort, which calls for increased nourishment, is difficult for the heart when the coronary arteries can't let through more blood.

Angina, as a rule, is felt as a constrictive sensation in the middle of the chest which often radiates, or shoots out, to the left arm and fingertips. But there are variations: occasionally, instead of in the chest, pain appears between the shoulder blades, in the left arm or shoulder, left hand or wrist, in the pit of the abdomen, in the jaws and teeth, or even in parts of the right arm.

Anginal chest pain has other characteristics. Usually, it is frightening as well as painful, triggering a sense of foreboding and compelling the victim to stop whatever he is doing.

Moreover, an attack is usually brief, over in a few minutes. It responds quickly to rest and, as well, to a nitroglycerin tablet. If chest pain persists for more than 15 minutes, it is not likely to be angina. You can be reassured that no heart attack is involved if the pain disappears quickly, but diagnosis by a physician is still warranted.

Heart Attack Chest Pain

The chest pain that is the hallmark of a heart attack can range from a slight feeling of pressure to a sensation that the chest is being crushed in a vise.

If an angina victim suffers a heart attack and at first assumes he is having just another angina attack, he should soon realize otherwise. This time, rest does no good, nor does nitroglycerin. Typically, the pain persists for hours and does not subside until a narcotic such as meperidine (Demerol) is administered.

Almost always with the chest pain there is grave anxiety, a

feeling that death is near. Commonly, the face turns ashen gray and a cold sweat appears. Often, retching, belching of gas, and vomiting develop and sometimes may make a victim think he is having a stomach upset. Shortness of breath is common. Sometimes, there may be palpitation—a sensation that the heart is beating abnormally fast and hard.

Some helps in distinguishing the chest pain of a heart attack from angina and from chest pains unrelated to the heart: It is less likely to be a heart attack if chest pain is below the nipple and to the left; if the pain is localized completely to the left; if the pain is sharp rather than a dull pressure or squeezing sensation; if the pain comes and goes; if the pain lessens when you lie down. If the pain persists for only one to five minutes, it is probably angina, not a heart attack.

What to Do for Angina

If you begin to experience what appear to be anginal chest pain attacks, based on the characteristics previously described, by all means see a physician for thorough examination and treatment.

Angina need not make an invalid of you nor seriously limit your activities. There are medications your physician can prescribe—nitroglycerin and others—which can be used safely and effectively not only to relieve angina but also to prevent recurrences. Other measures can help, including perhaps graduated exercise and change in diet and some practical changes in life-style.

What to Do for a Heart Attack

If you know—or even just suspect—you are having a heart attack, act promptly. The first hours and even minutes can sometimes be critical.

Ask someone to take you to the nearest hospital or call the rescue squad. And once you reach the emergency room, immediately tell personnel there that you may be having a heart attack and insist on being taken to the coronary care unit.

From the moment you suspect a heart attack, try to stay calm and avoid moving. Lie quietly; make no effort to get up or help yourself if help is on the way.

If you are with someone who seems to be having a heart attack, the most important thing you can do, once you have summoned medical help or are taking him to a hospital emergency room, is to talk to the victim quietly, providing reassurance, emphasizing that help is coming or he is on the way to it, and that he will be all right.

The fact is that while a heart attack can be immediately fatal, most attacks are not—and when a victim receives prompt medical care, the chances of getting well are very good.

Note: I have seen instances where an ambulance has reached a victim and very fine paramedics have done an electrocardiogram which has appeared to be normal and have then suggested that he remain at home. If this should happen in your case, don't accept the suggestion. Insist that you would rather be taken to the hospital and play it safe. Be happy the electrocardiogram is normal—but, should it change, you are better off in a hospital where you can be closely monitored and treated immediately.

Other Chest Pains Unrelated to the Heart

Once you have eliminated the possibility that sudden chest pain is related to the heart, it can be helpful for you—in deciding what the pain is coming from and what you should do for it—if you know a few basic facts about the chest and its contents.

The chest, of course, is the area of the body extending from below the neck to the *diaphragm*, the large flat muscle that separates chest from abdomen.

The chest is enclosed by the *rib cage*, consisting of twelve ribs and the muscles that join them together. Outside the ribs are muscles that move the cage and other muscles that move arms and shoulders.

Within the chest are the *lungs*, one on each side; the *heart*, which lies in the middle and extends a little toward the left; in the back, to the left and lying on the spine, the *aorta*, the

large vessel that emerges from the heart and distributes blood
to the entire body through arteries that branch from it; and,
lying slightly to the right side, the *esophagus*, a tube that is
part of the digestive system, about an inch in diameter, extending from throat to stomach, whose sole purpose is to carry
food and saliva from throat to stomach.

Lining the chest wall inside is a thin membrane, called the
pleura, similar in appearance to Saran Wrap. The lungs and
other organs within the chest are lined by a similar membrane.
There are no pain fibers in the membrane encasing the lungs
and other organs but there are in the pleura lining the chest
cavity, and this lining does cause pain if it is injured, irritated,
or inflamed.

PAIN FROM INJURY: This is common. Did you bump into
something, lift your child or grandchild a bit overexuberantly,
feel an unexpected twinge during a golf swing or tennis serve,
or perhaps get hit in the chest with a ball or other object?

If your chest pain—no matter where in the chest it is located
—is aching, dull, gnawing, and if moving the arms or bending
or sitting or standing or lying in a particular position is painful,
chances are your pain represents a bruised rib or a strain in
the muscles between the ribs (*intercostal muscles*) or in other
muscles attached to the chest wall that move the arm.

Take it easy for a time, giving the bruise or strain a chance
to heal, and you may need nothing more.

SHARP CHEST PAIN WITH A DEEP BREATH: If, on taking a
deep breath, you feel a sharp pain on either side of the chest,
this can be due to a fractured rib if there is a known injury
(see FRACTURES) or to pleurisy. With pleurisy, along with
sharp sticking chest pain, worse on inhaling, there may be
fever, cough, and chills (see PLEURISY).

SUDDEN SHARP CHEST PAIN EXTENDING TO A SHOULDER
OR DOWN OVER THE ABDOMEN: Such pain, accompanied by
breathing difficulty and sometimes, at the beginning, by a dry
hacking cough can indicate *pneumothorax,* collapse of a lung.
This occurs when air gets between the membrane lining the
chest wall and the membrane surrounding the lung, preventing the lung from expanding with each breath.

Pneumothorax can result from a knife or bullet wound, a car
accident, or other injury in which the chest is penetrated, al-

lowing air to enter. It can also occur spontaneously, for no special reason, or sometimes as the result of an existing lung disorder such as emphysema or, rarely, tuberculosis. Spontaneous pneumothorax also can be caused by rupture of a small balloonlike structure (a *bulla*) on a lung, which is most likely to occur in people with emphysema but also can happen in otherwise healthy people (most often in their teens and twenties). It has also occurred during diving and high-altitude flying.

There is a dangerous form of pneumothorax—the only type calling for emergency treatment—known as *tension pneumothorax*. In this, a tear in the pleura lets air in but not out, acting like a check valve. As pressure builds, the lung collapses completely, making breathing very difficult. Tension pneumothorax requires quick medical help, which can be lifesaving. Air must be removed and this may be done with needle and syringe. (See PNEUMOTHORAX.)

Air removal may be required in injury pneumothorax, along with treatment for the injury. A small spontaneous pneumothorax may require no special treatment; the air is reabsorbed in a few days. For a larger one, several weeks may be needed before all air is reabsorbed and the lung expands to normal; recovery may be speeded by treatment to remove the air. In any case, pneumothorax should have medical attention.

CHEST PAIN CAUSED BY THE ESOPHAGUS: Swallowing a hot liquid rapidly can cause chest pain because the heat is felt by nerves outside of the esophagus. Pain of an intermittent or chronic type can be caused by stomach acids "burning" the esophagus (see HEARTBURN).

CHEST PAIN FROM A RUPTURED ESOPHAGUS: This is a rare but critical cause of chest pain. Awareness of it is important, since the chances of cure depend upon how soon the condition is recognized and treatment carried out. Each hour counts. You can make the diagnosis by knowing the following: The rupture, or perforation, of the esophagus may result from severe vomiting or efforts to vomit (retching), straining at stool, swallowing a foreign object such as a meat or fish bone, or a crushing injury to the chest. Along with constantly worsening chest pain, there is breathlessness, and sometimes shock may develop. The perforation must be closed immediately by surgery and antibiotics administered to prevent serious infection.

HEART-ATTACKLIKE PAIN FROM A DISSECTING AORTIC ANEURYSM: An aneurysm is a dilation or ballooning out of part of a blood vessel, most often the aorta, the big trunkline artery emerging from the heart. In a dissecting aneurysm, the inner coat of the artery ruptures, permitting blood to enter between the layers of the artery wall, splitting or dissecting the wall.

Chest pain is severe, often mimicking the pain of a heart attack. A dissecting aortic aneurysm is usually the result of atherosclerosis and occurs mostly in older people. But it may result at any age from a severe accident such as slamming of the chest against a car steering wheel or a hard fall on the chest.

Hospitalization as quickly as possible is required. Medical treatment includes use of drugs to lower blood pressure. Surgical repair of the aorta may be needed.

OTHER CHEST PAIN: Chest pain can occur as one of many symptoms in infections, such as lung abscess (along with purulent sputum, cough, sweat, chills, and fever) or pneumonia (with pinkish sputum that may become rusty, fever, shaking chill, headache, rapid and painful breathing).

As a chronic rather than sudden acute problem, chest pain may occur in cancer of the lung and other lung disease such as silicosis.

Note, too: Chest pain can be part of the simple, yet often alarming condition of aerophagia, or excessive air swallowing, which also can produce abdominal distention, palpitation, breathing difficulty, smothering sensations, and other symptoms (see AIR SWALLOWING).

Choking on Food or a Foreign Object: Applying the Heimlich Maneuver

Choking is the sixth leading cause of accidental death and the leading cause in infants under age one in the home. It is sometimes called "cafe coronary" because in the past such deaths in restaurants often were confused with heart attacks.

It was in June, 1974, that *Emergency Medicine,* a publication for physicians, first published my description of a proposed method for saving the life of a person whose airway is obstructed by food or another foreign body.

The technique, to which others subsequently attached my name, is now known as the *Heimlich maneuver;* very quickly it received widespread recognition and use. In its first four years of use, several thousand lives have been reported saved. The technique is taught by many public and private organizations and agencies; more than 20 states have passed laws requiring that a description of the method be posted in eating establishments and in some instances also in schools. In some areas, state and county medical societies have induced food suppliers to print the details on milk cartons; and teaching programs have been instituted in many other countries.

The maneuver is *not* simply a first aid procedure. First aid is "what to do until the doctor arrives." Rather, the maneuver —or *Heimlich hug,* as it also is sometimes called—is a definitive treatment. It involves understanding how exactly to diagnose and know immediately when choking is occurring and how to treat immediately a condition that would otherwise be fatal within four minutes of onset. It is not possible for a mother at home or a choking diner in a restaurant to wait for a physician, paramedic, or ambulance.

For this reason, I hope you will read now, in advance of need, what follows. You can learn, quickly, the simple facts of both diagnosis and treatment.

Although the maneuver was originally conceived with the adult rescuer in mind, teaching of the technique in schools has resulted in children saving other children—and their parents.

In one instance, a mother was driving, with her children in the back seat, when she suddenly heard screams and turned around to see that one child was choking and had turned blue. She pulled over to the curb. By then, she found that her 8-year-old son was applying the maneuver to his 6-year-old brother; a piece of wax candy suddenly flew from the youngster's mouth and hit the windshield. The mother said she herself would not have known what to do.

In another instance, a 13-year-old, finding his choking

mother lying unconscious on the floor surrounded by his younger siblings, saved her by applying the maneuver in the supine position.

There have also been many reports of individuals who have saved themselves by self-application of the maneuver.

Diagnosis of Choking

Before the Heimlich maneuver brought public attention to the frequency of choking deaths, many persons choked to death while observers thought they were having heart attacks. There is no excuse for that now that the symptoms of choking have been defined. It is virtually impossible, knowing these symptoms, to think that a heart attack victim is choking. A heart attack victim is breathing and may complain of pain.

Besides, 25 percent of victims of choking are children, who are hardly likely to be suffering from heart attack. And 90 percent of choking victims are seen to be eating when choking occurs.

The setting is a clue—not only in but also near an eating place. It has been shown that over 98 percent of persons falling unconscious and dying in or near a restaurant or dining area have choked.

THE 1, 2, 3 OF RECOGNITION:

1. A person who is choking not only cannot breathe but also cannot speak, because the airway is blocked so no air can pass through the vocal cords.
2. A choking person turns blue, because oxygen is not reaching body tissues.
3. He falls unconscious, because oxygen is not reaching the brain.

In the various teaching programs for the maneuver used by public and other agencies, people are taught what has come to be known as the *Heimlich sign:* grasping the throat with the hand to indicate choking—a signal to a rescuer for prompt application of the maneuver. Once there is universal knowledge of the choking sign, diagnosis should be 100 percent.

When you see a person give the Heimlich sign, say "Are you choking?" If he nods his head yes, apply the maneuver.

But even without the sign, recognition of choking should not be a problem most of the time—in view of the inability of the victim to speak or breathe and the beginning of blueness even before the loss of consciousness that follows rapidly.

And even if an episode is not observed, anyone who is slumped over a chair or has fallen and is unconscious in or near any place where food is served is a candidate for the Heimlich maneuver. Delay, even to try CPR (see p. 52), may be fatal, as the unconscious choking victim is only seconds from death. Of course, if a person is unconscious, not in a dining area, and not breathing, the situation does not suggest choking and mouth-to-mouth resuscitation should be attempted immediately; any airway obstruction will be immediately obvious and the Heimlich maneuver should then be performed.

Basic Facts About the Maneuver

The maneuver avoids the problems with past approaches to handling choking. Inserting a finger or other object in the mouth in an effort to retrieve an obstructing piece of food or other item risks driving it farther down. Pounding on the back is inherently dangerous because it may wedge the material more deeply. The maneuver, as you will see, can drive the material only toward the mouth.

The basis for the maneuver is simple: Even in the midst of choking and inability to breathe, a great deal of air remains in the lungs—and if the lungs are properly compressed, the air can be driven out with enough force to pop the obstruction out of the throat and mouth.

That is exactly what the maneuver does. Actual laboratory trials with volunteers in which instrumentation was used to measure air flow, volume, and pressure have shown that when the maneuver is performed, it results in the expulsion of an average of about a quart (940 cc) of air from the mouth in a quarter of a second at an average pressure of 31 millimeters of mercury, sufficient to forcefully eject an object partially or totally obstructing the airway.

The maneuver can be performed when the victim is standing, sitting, or lying on his back. And you can perform it on yourself if that should ever be necessary.

How to Perform the Heimlich Maneuver

STANDING POSITION: Stand behind the victim.

1. Wrap your arms around his waist.
2. Make a fist and place the thumb side against the victim's abdomen—*slightly above* the navel or belly button and *below* the rib cage.
3. Grasp your fist with your other hand and press into the victim's abdomen with a *quick upward thrust.* Repeat several times if necessary.

Note carefully: You press your fist into the abdomen below the rib cage by bending your arm at the elbow. Do not squeeze or compress the chest; this can cause serious injuries. I like to emphasize this instruction by saying, "The victim's life is in your *hands!*" (Not in your arms.) A review from the Mayo Clinic noted that with CPR—which, unlike the Heimlich maneuver, requires pressure on the rib cage—ribs have been fractured and chests crushed, causing fatal internal injuries.

SITTING POSITION: When the victim is sitting, stand or kneel behind his chair and perform the maneuver exactly as for the standing position.

LYING ON THE BACK (SUPINE POSITION): When a victim has fallen, don't waste time trying to elevate him to standing or sitting position. Turn him on his back, with face upward, if he is not already in that position.

1. Face the victim's face, and kneel astride his hips.
2. With one of your hands on top of the other, place the *heel* of your bottom hand (the part of the hand hear the wrist) on the victim's abdomen, slightly above the navel and below the rib cage.
3. Press into the victim's abdomen with a *quick upward thrust.* Repeat several times if necessary.

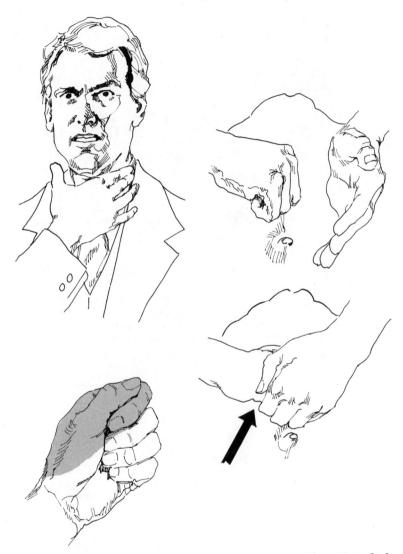

Fig. 1. Heimlich Maneuver. UPPER LEFT: The Heimlich sign. Hand to neck indicates: "I am choking!" LOWER LEFT: Making the fist (shaded area indicates "knob" to be used for pressing into abdomen). UPPER RIGHT: Placement of fist on abdomen. LOWER RIGHT: Position of other hand.

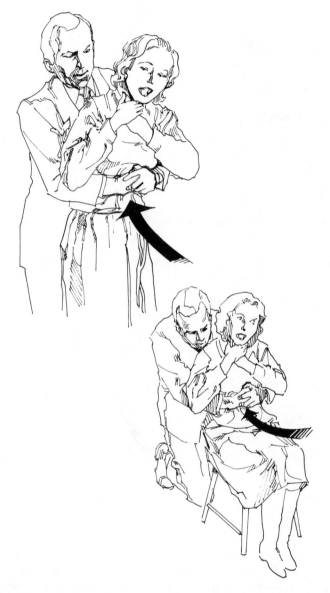

Fig. 2. Heimlich Maneuver. TOP: For a standing victim. BOTTOM: For a seated victim.

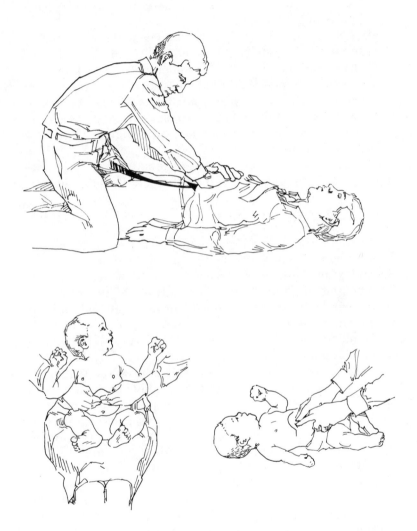

Fig. 3. Heimlich Maneuver. TOP: For a fallen victim or a small rescuer saving a husky victim. The rescuer uses his own body weight to perform the Maneuver. BOTTOM: For an infant.

SELF-ADMINISTERING THE MANEUVER: If you yourself are choking and no one is present to help, you can perform the maneuver on yourself. Many people, aged 10 years to 85, have saved their own lives in this manner.

Place the thumb side of your fist into your abdomen, below the ribs and slightly above the navel. Grasp your fist with your other hand and press into the abdomen with a quick upward thrust exactly as you would do if you were attempting to save someone else. Or you can lean your abdomen against the back or edge of a chair, sink, table, even porch rail and press against it, applying pressure in the same place, slightly above the navel and beneath the rib cage.

SPECIAL NOTES: In 90 percent of reported cases, the maneuver has been applied from behind the victim, who was standing or sitting.

There are, however, two specific situations in which the supine, or lying-on-the-back, position is essential. First, as already noted, if the choking victim is unconscious and on the floor, no time should be wasted trying to stand or sit him up. Second, if the rescuer is too small or weak to reach around from behind, or if the victim is markedly obese, the maneuver can be performed only with the victim supine. Children have saved parents in the supine position, and petite wives their husky husbands.

It is essential in every case that the rescuer kneel astride a supine victim—never alongside—so that he can press into the middle of the abdomen and use the weight of his own body to apply enough pressure to elevate the diaphragm and compress the lungs quickly. Not only is the upward thrust less effective from the side of the victim, but it is impossible to apply the thrust directly in the midline. Inadvertent pressure to either side of the abdomen could rupture the liver or the spleen.

It is also essential, when using the maneuver on a supine victim, that his face be looking up; if the head is turned to one side (as may be necessary in other circumstances to prevent getting vomitus, blood, or water into the lungs, the throat will be contorted and a solid object obstructing the airway will not be able to pass through. If vomiting does follow the performance of the maneuver, you can then turn the victim's head to the side and wipe out the mouth.

For the Infant Victim: There are two ways to apply the maneuver to an infant.

You can hold him seated in your lap. Reach around and place the index and middle fingers of both hands against the baby's abdomen, above the navel and below the rib cage. Then press into the abdomen with a quick upward thrust.

Or you can place the infant face upward on a firm surface and perform the maneuver while facing him, again using index and middle fingers of both hands.

Common sense tells you to be gentle when performing the maneuver on an infant.

Artificial Respiration—When Breathing Has Stopped

Breathing failure has many possible causes, including drowning, electric shock, drug poisoning, chemical fumes, blocking of the airway by a foreign object, acute asthma, croup, and medical shock.

What to Do: Examine the victim's mouth and throat; remove any foreign matter.

Check for any indications of breathing: movement of chest, air coming from nose or mouth. Check the wrist for a pulse. If there is neither breathing nor pulse, go to CPR (cardiopulmonary resuscitation). If the victim is not breathing but you feel a pulse, indicating the heart is still beating, apply mouth-to-mouth artificial respiration:

1. Lay the victim on his back. Place one hand under his neck, lift up on the neck, use the heel of your other hand on his forehead to tilt the head back, thus opening the air passage.

2. Put your mouth, wide open, around the victim's open mouth, pinch his nostrils shut, and blow hard enough so his chest rises. If a small child is the victim, place your mouth over the child's mouth *and* nose while blowing.

3. When the victim's chest has expanded, stop blowing, remove your mouth, listen for the sound of exhaled air, and look for the chest to fall. Repeat the blowing and exhalation cycle.

4. If there is no air exchange, check the victim's mouth again. His tongue may be blocking the air passage. If there is still no air exchange, a foreign body deep in the air passage may be causing obstruction. With the victim still on his back, face upward, kneel astride his hips facing him, and use the Heimlich maneuver to expel the object. To do this, place one of your hands on top the other, set the heel of the bottom hand on the abdomen, slightly above the navel or bellybutton and below the rib cage. Press into the abdomen with a quick upward thrust. Repeat several times.

5. After the foreign body has been expelled, if the victim still is not breathing, begin mouth-to-mouth breathing again. Blow one vigorous breath every five seconds for an adult. For a child, blow smaller, less vigorous breaths every three seconds.

6. Don't stop. Keep up the artificial respiration until the victim begins to breathe. Many people have resumed breathing after several hours.

7. Have a physician or ambulance summoned as soon as you can. When breathing resumes, use blankets or coats under and over the victim to keep him warm.

Note: Many thousands of people have had surgical removal of part or all of their larynxes. They cannot use nose or mouth for breathing; instead, they breathe through an opening (stoma) in the windpipe in front of the neck.

When trying to help a victim of an accident or sudden illness, examine the front of the neck to see if there is an opening there (in some cases, a breathing tube may be worn in the stoma; if so, leave it in place unless it becomes clogged).

Use the same procedure as for mouth-to-mouth resuscitation but place your mouth over the stoma. There is often no need in this case to tilt the head back or to close off the nose and mouth. If, however, the chest does not rise when you blow through the stoma and the stoma is clear, the larynx removal may have been only partial and the victim may normally breathe through both stoma *and* mouth and nose. Tilt the victim's head back, close off mouth and nose, and blow again through the stoma.

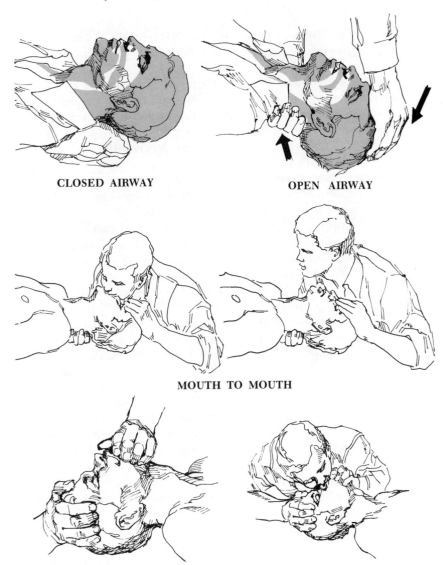

CLOSED AIRWAY   OPEN AIRWAY

MOUTH TO MOUTH

MOUTH TO NOSE

Fig. 4. Cardiopulmonary resuscitation. TOP: Establishing an open airway. MIDDLE: Mouth-to-mouth breathing. BOTTOM: Mouth-to-nose breathing.

CPR (Cardiopulmonary Resuscitation)—When Breathing and Heart Stop

CPR, meant for use when there is no breathing and the heart has stopped (as indicated by lack of pulse), includes closed-chest heart massage as well as mouth-to-mouth respiration.

CPR can be lifesaving. But if used unnecessarily and incorrectly it can be devastating.

Closed-chest heart massage always carries some degree of risk of causing serious internal injuries—by crushing the chest or fracturing ribs that may puncture lungs, liver, stomach, or spleen. The risk is very much worth taking when CPR is essential in a situation where life otherwise will be lost.

The risk is greatly reduced when the procedure is applied expertly by someone who has had training through a special course in which there is manikin practice. Such a course provides skill that cannot be imparted in a book. But information on CPR is provided here for desperate emergency use.

Please note: Don't mistake unconsciousness from a faint, choking, diabetic coma, or other condition for heart and breathing arrest. It could be tragic to use CPR and cause injury —especially if you are not expert in its use—in such conditions for which it is of no value. If you are in or adjacent to a dining area, there is a 98 percent chance that the unconscious victim has choked on food, and you must immediately do the Heimlich maneuver. *Do now read* carefully the previous sections on CHOKING and POISONING and the later sections on FAINTNESS AND FAINTING, DIABETIC REACTIONS, STROKE, also the information on skull fracture in the section on FRACTURES, DISLOCATIONS, SPRAINS AND STRAINS.

WHAT TO DO: After first making certain there is neither breathing nor heartbeat (no pulse at the wrist), quickly check the victim's mouth and throat and remove any foreign matter.

Then you and someone to assist you—or you alone, if necessary—proceed thus:

1. Lay the victim on his back. Kneeling at his side, strike your fist sharply down on his breastbone. This may start the

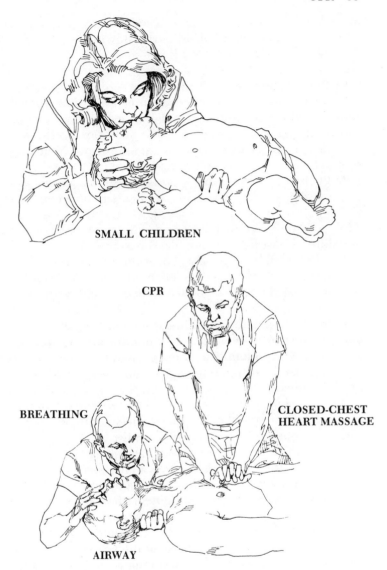

SMALL CHILDREN

CPR

BREATHING

CLOSED-CHEST HEART MASSAGE

AIRWAY

Fig. 5. Cardiopulmonary resuscitation. TOP: Mouth-to-mouth-and-nose breathing for a small child. BOTTOM: Mouth-to-mouth breathing and closed-chest heart massage.

heart beating. (*Note:* This step, used for any purpose other than instituting a normal heart beat following heart stoppage, can severely injure the heart.) If not——

2. Feel the victim's chest to locate the lower tip of the breastbone. Pressure must not be applied here or the liver may be injured. Instead, find a point three fingerbreadths above the tip of the breastbone. Place one finger at that point and position the heel of the second hand next to the finger. Then place the heel of the first hand on top. Your fingers should be intertwined and lifted off the chest.

3. Push down with a quick thrust, using the weight of the upper part of your body to achieve sufficient force to press the lower portion of the breastbone down 1½ to 2 inches in an adult. Then lift your weight. The downward pressure acts as a heartbeat substitute, pushing blood out from the heart to circulate through the body. Repeat the compression rhythmically once a second. If you have not been trained in the technique, remember, again, the danger of crushing the chest if you press too hard.

4. Mouth-to-mouth breathing also must be used. If you have no one to assist you, give 15 chest compressions and then stop in order to administer 2 deep mouth-to-mouth breaths. Keep up the 15 compressions to 2 mouth-to-mouth breaths until help arrives.

If an assistant is available, have him administer mouth-to-mouth respiration at the rate of 12 times a minute—once for every 5 compressions that you administer.

5. Continue the complete CPR (chest compression and mouth-to-mouth breathing) until the victim begins to breathe, pulse returns, and color improves. Do *not* give up after just a few minutes. Life can be maintained by CPR for an hour or more.

Note: If you would like to become expert in administering CPR, courses of instruction may be offered in your community. I cannot vouch for the success of CPR because the reports of its use are confusing. The method is reported here because it is so widely talked about, and its mention here does not necessarily indicate that I endorse its use.

Burns

Burns can range from the relatively trivial, even if painful, to the devastating and life-threatening. And there are three factors to consider in determining how serious a burn is, what treatment to use, and whether medical attention is urgent. Those factors are

1. The class or degree of burn—essentially, a matter of depth
2. The extent—how much area is involved
3. The location

DEGREES: In a *first*-degree burn—which may result from sun exposure, light contact with a hot object, or brief scalding by hot water or steam—only the outer surface of the skin is involved. The skin is red, dry, painful, sensitive to touch, mildly swollen.

A *second*-degree burn produces redness or mottling, blisters, weeping and wetness, swelling, and pain. The burn has penetrated deeper into lower layers of the skin. The blistering results from bubbling of blood plasma through the damaged layers. A second-degree burn may result from severe sunburn, a flash from gasoline or kerosene, a spill of boiling water on the skin.

A *third*-degree burn involves not only the outer and deeper layers of the skin but also tissue below the skin. The skin is usually either pale white or charred black. It is swollen. Often underlying tissues are exposed. A third-degree burn may result when clothes are ignited or there is exposure to a flame, an electrical current, or hot object. Length of exposure and degree of heat are important in determining the amount of tissue destroyed. Often, because pain nerves are destroyed, there may be no severe local pain in the burn area, but the margin of the burn may be painful.

EXTENT OF BURN: Determining the extent is important because in an adult who suffers burns of 15 percent or more of the body surface—in a child, 10 percent or more—there is

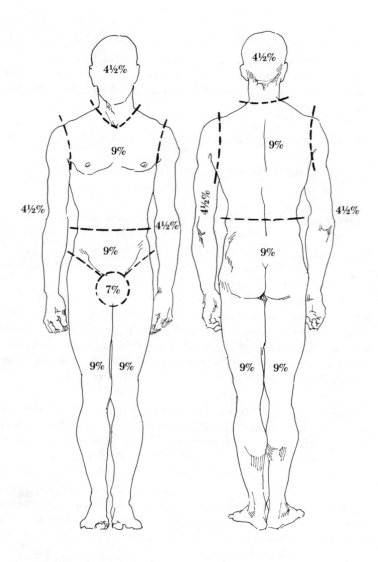

Fig. 6. Determining extent of burns. Numbers indicate the proportion of various body regions to total skin area.

likely to be shock (see previous section on SHOCK). Any burned person showing symptoms of impending shock should be taken to a hospital.

You can roughly estimate the extent of a burn in this way: Figure that the surface area of a hand (both sides) equals about 1 percent of total skin area. Alternatively, you can figure that in an average adult, the head has 9 percent of total skin surface; each arm, 9 percent; each leg, 18 percent; front and back of the trunk, 18 percent each; neck, 1 percent.

LOCATION: When the face is burned, there may be injury to the breathing passages, and as respiratory tissues swell, breathing may become obstructed. If the victim has difficulty speaking, swallowing or breathing, or is hoarse or wheezing, hospitalization is usually needed.

Burns involving the area around the eyes should be examined immediately by an eye doctor.

Second- or third-degree burns of the hand or any joint (elbow, knee, shoulder, etc.) should always be seen by a physician because contracting scars can develop later and interfere with function and movement.

WHAT TO DO: Remove clothing over the burned area immediately to prevent further burning.

For a first-degree burn, apply cold water or immerse the burned area in cold water. If the burn is dirty, wash gently with soapy water, then flush with large amounts of cold water. Cooling can provide substantial relief and may speed recovery. If necessary, apply a dry dressing. If no complications occur, a first-degree burn should be comfortable within 12 to 24 hours and healed in about a week.

For a second-degree burn, immerse the burned area in cold water until pain subsides. Apply clean cloths wrung out in ice water for as long as an hour. Then gently blot the area dry. Do *not* break blisters and do *not* apply antiseptic sprays, ointments, etc. Apply a layer of nonadherent, light impregnated gauze such as sterile petrolatum gauze (obtainable in most drugstores) and hold in place with dry sterile gauze and a loosely wrapped bandage. If an arm or leg is burned, keep it elevated. Change the dressing next day and about every two days after that. If fever develops or if pain and swelling increase, an infection is likely to be present and antibiotic treatment may be necessary. A physician should be consulted.

For a third-degree burn, medical help is needed immediately. Infection may set in, healing is slow, scars can occur, and surgery may be required. Usually, too, intravenous fluids and treatment for shock are needed.

If the victim of a third-degree burn can be transported to a hospital immediately or medical help will arrive very quickly, make the victim as comfortable as possible. If the hands are burned, keep them above the level of the heart; elevate burned feet or legs. If the face is burned, prop up the victim and watch continuously for any breathing difficulty; if any develops, maintain an open airway (see p. 50).

If medical help will be delayed, remove clothing but do not remove any adhered particles of charred garments. Do *not* apply ointments, grease, other remedies or commercial preparations. Cover the burn with sterile dressings of clean household linen. You may simply have the patient lie on a clean sheet and loosely cover him with a second sheet.

Do *not* apply ice water to or immerse a large burned area; that may intensify shock. But a cold pack can be used on the face.

If the victim is conscious and not vomiting, have him slowly sip a weak solution of salt and soda, neither hot nor cold, made with one level teaspoonful of table salt and one-half level teaspoonful of baking soda to a quart of water. Give about half a glass over a 15-minute period to an adult, a quarter glass to a child, about an eighth glass to an infant. Stop fluid if vomiting occurs.

Chemical Burns

Of the skin: As quickly as possible, wash away the chemical with water, large quantities of it. Use a hose spray or shower if you can. Remove clothing from involved area and continue flushing with water for at least five minutes. If there is a container of the chemical with first aid directions for that particular chemical, follow them after the water flushing. Apply a clean dry bandage and get medical help.

Of the eye: Every part of the body is important, but few if any tragedies are greater than the unnecessary loss of an eye. Accidental splashing of a chemical into an eye is a danger in a chemical laboratory—but it can also occur in the home. I recall a woman who poured a drain cleaner (lye) into her kitchen sink. It generated heat and pressure, shooting upward into her eye.

As quickly as possible, pour warm but not hot tap water from a pitcher into the eye, with head tilted backward. To do this successfully, you may have to hold the eye open with the thumb and forefinger of one hand. It does no good to pour the water on a closed lid. Hold the pitcher close to the eye to obtain a gentle flow. If it is held too high, the pressure of the water could cause damage. Continue this flushing for five minutes, and without delay arrange for transportation to an eye doctor. In the meantime, after the flushing, cover the closed eye with clean, dry dressing and bandage. *Do not rub the eye.*

Save That Accidentally Amputated Body Part

At 6 A.M. on a September morning in San Francisco, a housewife was awakened from sleep by screams outside her window. It was a garbage-collection morning in the neighborhood. The truck had stopped at her door. In a cruel moment, the left hand of one of the collection crew became caught in the truck's compressor mechanism and was torn away.

When she called from her window to find out what was wrong, the man held his arm up and she could see that his hand was gone. The housewife quickly phoned for an ambulance. While her husband took down some towels for the other men to wrap around the young man's arm, she went to her kitchen and got a plastic bag and some ice cubes, intending to get the hand and put it into the bag.

But the hand had gone inside the truck. As the driver of the truck let some of the garbage down into the street, she shoved the trash around with a broom. After three minutes, she found the hand, still in a glove, and placed it in the bag of ice. When the ambulance arrived, she gave the bag to the attendant.

At that point, she went into the house and prayed.

Not long afterward, at San Francisco General Hospital, surgeons began an operation that lasted ten hours. Working precisely under microscopes, they realigned bones and reconnected muscles, tissue, tendons, blood vessels, and nerves. Because the hand arrived with the patient, the reconnection could begin within two hours of the accident. And because the hand had been packed in ice, onset of deterioration had been stalled. Today, the grateful victim has two hands.

Perhaps of all accidents, those involving amputations are most distressing. But cool thinking, exemplified in this case, can make a vital, rewarding difference now that surgical techniques have advanced to the point of often allowing the grafting back of severed body parts.

If you should ever be faced with such a situation, do exactly what the San Francisco housewife did:

1. Call for, or get the victim to, medical help.
2. Preserve the amputated part, if possible packed in ice. Whether it's a finger, arm, leg, ear, tip of nose, keeping the part cold cuts down the need for oxygen and extends the life of the part as long as four hours.
3. Make certain it accompanies the victim to medical help.

Note, too: If your child should have a permanent tooth accidentally knocked out, or if you yourself should be the victim, there is a good chance that it can be reimplanted successfully if you act promptly (see TOOTH, KNOCKED-OUT).

Coughing

Coughing has a purpose. It's an attempt by the body to get rid of materials—fluids, mucus, dust, other substances—from the lungs, windpipe, or throat where they don't belong. An effective cough can be a powerful force, releasing a burst of air at speeds of as much as 500 feet per second.

Because coughing is often protective, it is not always wise to try to suppress it with anticough medication.

And, in fact, it can be helpful for you to know how to work with your cough—to make it, if necessary, more protective.

SUDDEN COUGH: Commonly, a cough that comes on suddenly does so because food or liquid has accidentally started down the wrong way into the lungs instead of the stomach. The food irritates the lining of the airway, triggering a cough as a natural protective mechanism.

Normally, when you swallow, several things happen automatically. The opening of the airway to the lungs, called the *glottis*, lies just behind and below the tongue. And right above the glottis is a flaplike structure called the *epiglottis*, which is attached to the root of the tongue.

With normal swallowing, the glottis instantly moves under the epiglottis so the flap of tissue can seal it off (much in the manner in which a flap valve closes), thus barring entrance of food or liquid into the airway, leaving open only the food passage. So securely in fact is the airway sealed off that if you were to try to stop halfway in the act of swallowing to take a breath, you would find yourself unable to breathe until you complete the swallowing act.

But accidents happen. Occasionally, you swallow the wrong way—which is to say that the epiglottis fails to function effectively, possibly because you were talking, laughing, or eating too fast. A bite of food or a swallow of liquid then moves into the glottis and you cough explosively to blow the material out.

It's important that the foreign material be expelled, because if it were to reach a lung, it could damage lung tissue or cause lung infection.

The best thing to do when a cough comes on under such circumstances is to encourage it—and, if necessary, make it more effective when, as sometimes happens, it becomes violent but not effective.

So you need to know the simple steps involved in producing an effective cough.

The first step is breathing in deeply to get a large quantity of air into the lungs. Then, the opening of the glottis to the airway is closed as it moves under the epiglottis. Now, for a fraction of a second, you stop breathing and the diaphragm and muscles of your chest wall are splinted or held still. Try this—holding your breath purposely by compressing the muscles of your chest as if to blow air out but tightening your throat to keep the air from coming out. (This is what a child does when he has a temper tantrum and holds his breath.)

In the next step, the chest wall muscles are suddenly contracted further, reducing the inner volume of the chest and compressing the lungs. At this moment, the glottis opens and air suddenly rushes out.

That's the process involved in coughing.

If you find that your automatic coughing is not effectively eliminating a foreign object in your throat or windpipe, take a very deep breath and give a deep forceful cough, feeling it come up from the diaphragm. To be most effective, try to breathe in deeply enough to be able to cough out two or three times in succession without taking a second breath.

CHRONIC COUGH: A chronic cough that is not effective can be disturbing as well as useless.

Let's say that your chronic cough is associated with bronchitis or pneumonia. There may then be much mucus in the lungs and air passages. The mucous membrane lining in the passages secretes a sticky fluid, *mucus,* which serves to trap dust and other particles in inhaled air. Also in the passages are microscopic, hairlike projections called *cilia.* The cilia, through a continuous whiplike motion in the direction of the mouth, carry the sticky fluid upward so it can be swallowed or expectorated, thus helping to keep the air passages and lungs clean.

When mucus is excessive, the cilia may not be able to keep up, and the mucus must be eliminated by coughing. Similarly, the cilia may not be able to cope adequately if you have postnasal drip and secretions from the sinuses drain down the back of the throat and into the bronchial passages.

So if you have an accumulation of mucus and your coughing, though chronic and repeated, is not bringing the mucus up effectively, go through the cough procedure noted above and your coughing may become effective. Steam inhalation often can be helpful, too, by decreasing the viscosity or stickiness of the secretions so they become easier to bring up.

By all means, do not be finicky about coughing up and expectorating mucus into a paper tissue. That's where it belongs, not down in your lungs and breathing passages, and, in fact, it is not healthy to swallow excessive mucus.

COUGHING BLOOD: Sometimes, after a violent sudden fit of coughing or with chronic coughing associated with a cold, allergy or bronchitis, you may see a small fleck of bright red or brownish blood in the sputum.

This is not unusual and need not be alarming. The strain of coughing and/or the irritation of the airways caused by infection or inflammation can produce the same type of abrasive effect on the linings of the breathing passages as would scraping some skin off the surface of an arm, in which case you would also see a small amount of blood.

If, however, there is more than one episode of coughing up a small amount of blood, it would be wise to see your physician for studies that may include a chest x-ray. He may also perform *bronchoscopy*, using a lighted instrument to examine the air passages. Bronchoscopy, formerly somewhat difficult because a rigid metal tube was used, now is done with a very small flexible fiberoptic instrument and hospitalization is not necessary.

If you cough up a fair amount of blood—say, the equivalent of a teaspoonful of pure blood or more—that can indicate a possibly serious underlying condition; it may, for example, be the first indication of lung disease. Even though it is a first episode and occurs only that once, you should consult your physician about it, not necessarily as an emergency condition calling for immediate attention, but by the next morning if it occurs at night.

If you cough up a great deal of blood or repeated modest amounts, emergency medical treatment is needed. Try to determine, if possible, where the blood is coming from— whether from the lungs, from vomiting, or has come up from the stomach to the throat and been coughed up. This information will help your physician to initiate the proper tests and treatment.

Note: Sometimes, coughing up of a sizable amount of blood can be due to a nosebleed that occurs during the night and is not noticed while you are sleeping. When you wake, you may

cough up the blood from the nosebleed. Similarly, a nosebleed that occurs while you are awake may sometimes cause
blood to run down the back of the throat and be coughed up.
Such coughing up of blood is relatively rare. Stop the nosebleed (see BLEEDING FROM THE NOSE) and have the cause
checked out by a physician.

Medical Emergency Kits

Remember the last time someone in the family cut a finger
or picked up a splinter, or your visiting Aunt Lizzie tripped on
a step—and you hunted fruitlessly in the medicine cabinet
jumble for needed supplies and had to end up rushing off to
the drugstore?

Yours will have been no isolated experience.

Supplies for medical emergencies don't have to take up
great space—but they deserve their own space. Take the time
to assemble those supplies, before you need them. Do this
now!

I am presenting here suggestions for basic kits for the home
and for the car and suggestions, too, for what to take with you
for ordinary travel and also for a hunting, fishing, or other trips
which may take you where medical help may not be close at
hand.

Except where specifically noted otherwise, the suggested
items can be obtained without prescription.

You should not put your home supplies in with other items
in the medicine cabinet. Instead, keep them separately in a
labeled container, which can be an old tackle box or small tool
chest with hinged cover, or anything else suitable. Keep emergency supplies for the car in a similar container.

Keep the home container unlocked, on a shelf beyond a tot's
reach.

Basic Home Kit

Sterile gauze dressings, individually wrapped, in 2- x 2-inch
and 4- x 4-inch sizes, for cleaning and covering wounds

Piece of an old bedsheet, clean, folded, for use in making bandages and slings and in tying on splints

Roll of 2-inch gauze bandage, for securing dressings over wounds

Roll of half-inch-wide adhesive tape

Cotton applicators, small package, for removing foreign body from the eye

Feminine napkins, four, useful for staunching heavy bleeding anywhere on the body

Rubbing alcohol (isopropyl, 70%), small bottle, for sterilizing instruments and for sponging the body during high fever

Calamine lotion, small bottle, for insect bites, rashes, sunburn, etc.

Syrup of ipecac, 1 oz bottle, to induce vomiting in case of poisoning

Activated charcoal, useful for flatulence (gas)

Tube of petroleum jelly (petrolatum)

Band-Aids or equivalent, assorted sizes

Aromatic spirits of ammonia, small bottle

Aspirin or acetaminophen

Mild, nonstinging antiseptic such as Merthiolate, Zephiran Chloride, or Betadine

Milk of magnesia

Rectal and oral thermometers

Tweezers

Scissors with blunt tips, for cutting tape and gauze

Thick, blunt needle for removing splinters

Tongue depressors, for small splints

Basic Kit for the Car

Table salt and baking soda, 1 small package each

Matches, box

Bottle of distilled water, for burns and washing wounds

Sterile gauze dressings, individually wrapped, in 2- x 2-inch and 4- x 4-inch size

Piece of an old bedsheet, clean, folded

Roll of 2-inch gauze bandage

Roll of half-inch-wide adhesive tape

Cotton applicators, small package

Feminine napkins, four
Rubbing alcohol
Tube of petroleum jelly (petrolatum)
Band-Aids or equivalent, assorted sizes
Aromatic spirits of ammonia, small bottle
Aspirin or acetaminophen
Mild, nonstinging antiseptic such as Merthiolate, Zephiran
   Chloride, or Betadine
Tweezers
Scissors with blunt tips
Thick, blunt needle

Basic Kit for Travel

Steristrips, for use (instead of sutures) in holding together the
   cut edges of a laceration
Oral antibiotic for infections, prescribed by your physician
Dramamine tablets, for motion sickness
Emetrol, for nausea and vomiting
Kaopectate, for diarrhea
Pepto-Bismol, for treatment and prevention of traveler's diar-
   rhea (turista) if you go to a developing country
Doxycycline, an antibiotic your physician can prescribe, for
   preventing diarrhea (turista) if you go to a developing coun-
   try
Sterile gauze dressings, individually wrapped, 2- x 2-inch and
   4- x 4-inch sizes
Roll of 2-inch gauze bandage
Roll of half-inch-wide adhesive tape
Cotton applicators, small package
Tube of petroleum jelly (petrolatum)
Rectal and oral thermometers
Aromatic spirits of ammonia, small bottle
Tweezers
Band-Aids or equivalent, assorted sizes
Aspirin or acetaminophen
(If you use reading glasses, it would be advisable to take
   along, in case of loss, inexpensive eyeglasses with simple
   magnifying lenses, obtainable at "five-and-dime" and other
   stores)

Basic Kit for Travel to Isolated Areas

In addition to the items just listed for ordinary travel, it would be wise to add:

Snakebite kit

Suturing equipment

ABOUT SUTURING EQUIPMENT AND SUTURING: It would be advisable to check with your physician for additional advice and perhaps some basic instruction he may be willing to give you.

A sterile suture package is available, with nylon thread joined to the end of a needle. Size 3-0 suture thread is generally useful except for the face; 5-0, which is finer, is less likely to leave a scar.

The needle can be held with a *hemostat*—a clamplike instrument that amounts to a small, self-locking, needle-nosed plier, which also has some usefulness in removing thorns and fishhooks, and even on occasion for repairing fishing and other equipment.

Suturing may be necessary only when a wound gapes so much that it cannot be treated any other way. In most cases, but not all, the wound edges can be brought together and held with a Steristrip. A deep cut in an area of the body subject to much movement sometimes can be a problem.

When suturing appears to be essential, clean the wound with soap and water, then dry it.

Holding the needle with the hemostat, take a stitch through the skin only, never beyond into fat or muscle. The skin is never more than a quarter of an inch thick. By staying within the skin, you penetrate no vital structure. If you should hit a blood vessel, pull the suture through and out, and start again in a site just a little above or below. Bleeding will stop if you apply pressure for a minute or so.

After taking the stitch, tie the thread with three knots. Cut off the extra thread, leaving the stitch ends about a quarter of an inch long to help remove them in about seven days.

Although there is some pain during suturing, it is not agonizing and lasts for only a second or two.

Avoid suturing near an eyelid since the skin may be distorted during healing, causing trouble later.

Part Two

A Complete, Alphabetical, Cross-Referenced Guide to Emergency Medical Situations

Fig. 7. The gastro-
intestinal tract.

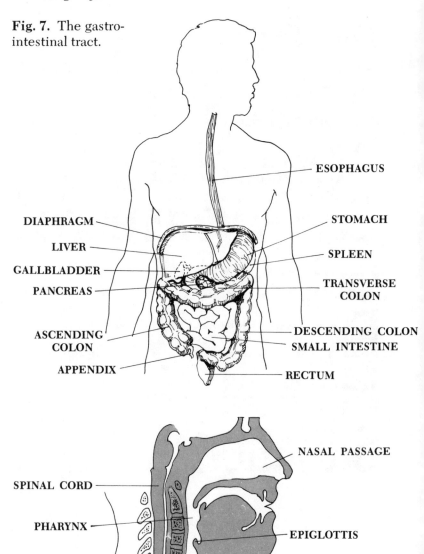

ESOPHAGUS

DIAPHRAGM

STOMACH

LIVER

SPLEEN

GALLBLADDER

TRANSVERSE
COLON

PANCREAS

ASCENDING
COLON

DESCENDING COLON

SMALL INTESTINE

APPENDIX

RECTUM

NASAL PASSAGE

SPINAL CORD

PHARYNX

EPIGLOTTIS

VERTEBRAL
COLUMN

ESOPHAGUS

TRACHEA

Fig. 8. Breathing and swallowing passages.

Abrasions (Scrapes)

These skin wounds, usually the result of scraping or rubbing, are shallow and do not go below the skin. But they can be painful, sometimes more so than cuts. Often, in addition to oozing of blood, many nerve endings are exposed, which is why the pain is severe.

WHAT TO DO: Take care to remove any splinters or foreign objects that may be embedded in the skin—and to guard against infection.

For removing objects, clean tweezers (dipped in alcohol for five minutes) are useful.

Thoroughly wash the wound with warm water and soap; this is most important. A bath or shower may be the best way to cleanse the wound.

You can cover with a sterile dressing if the wound is extensive, but this is not often necessary unless there is continued oozing of blood. It is best to use a nonadherent dressing—one that will not stick to the open area of skin.

If infection develops, it will not necessarily be obvious for 24 hours or so. Keep an eye out for any fever, pus, marked swelling, or redness. Swollen, tender glands (lymph nodes) in the armpit or groin also indicate infection. Redness about the edges of the abrasion is no cause for alarm but is part of the normal healing process.

If infection does develop, see a physician. Also see a physician if you are unable to get all the debris out from under the skin since, if left, it may lead to permanent discoloration. If the abrasion is extensive, and especially if there is debris under the skin, a tetanus injection may be wise.

Adhesions (See INTESTINAL OBSTRUCTION)

Air Swallowing (Aerophagia)

Aerophagia, or habitual swallowing of air, can when extreme produce alarming symptoms including abdominal distention, cramps, breathing difficulty, smothering sensations, palpitations, or seeming heart pain.

A little air, of no consequence, is unavoidably swallowed with food. But large, disturbing amounts may be swallowed by anyone who eats rapidly or eats while emotionally upset. Often, the victim is unaware of the air swallowing.

Much air also can be swallowed in drinking large amounts of carbonated beverages, during smoking, and during gum chewing. Some people just swallow air from habit when nervous.

If, after swallowing much air, you remain in upright position, the air, upon arriving in the stomach, rises above the stomach's liquid contents, comes in contact with the stomach's junction with the esophagus, or gullet, and is belched. Belching, however, may get rid of some air only to take in more if the mouth is kept closed. When you're in supine position (lying on your back), swallowed air is trapped below the fluid in the stomach and is often propelled into the intestines.

WHAT TO DO: To overcome an aerophagic habit, you may have to avoid candy mints, gum, carbonated drinks, rapid eating, and even excessively animated mealtime conversations that can lead to food gulping and much air swallowing.

To get relief from a lot of swallowed air which has moved into the intestines and may not be moving on from there well enough or rapidly enough to avoid "gas" and its symptoms, try the measures suggested under FLATULENCE.

Air-Travel Ankle Swelling

Ankle swelling during a long airplane flight is a relatively common problem. The cause appears to be prolonged sitting, with the upward pressure of the seat and unrelieved bending of the knee reducing blood circulation, allowing fluid to accumulate in tissues, leading to edema with ankle swelling.

Under ordinary circumstances, the movement of leg muscles produces a pumplike effect that helps move blood upward from the legs to the heart. Even the comparatively little leg muscle movement that is carried out during a train or car ride seems enough to maintain circulation.

WHAT TO DO: As a means of both treating and preventing airplane ankle, exercise at least the toes and ankles briefly every half hour while on a plane and, if possible, get up and walk about for brief periods. If confined to your seat, make bicycle-riding motions, using thigh, knee, leg, ankle and foot, one side at a time. Should your seatmates think you are peculiar, explain what you are doing. I'm sure they will shortly be joining you in the exercises.

Air-Travel Ear/Sinus Pain

With aircraft cabins pressurized, fewer air travelers now experience ear or sinus difficulties. When such problems do occur, they usually appear during descent.

Ear Pain

In what is called *barotitis media*, pain and some temporary hearing loss occur. This is most likely to happen if you have a cold or other upper respiratory infection. Then, the throat openings of the eustachian tubes, which lead to the ears, may be inflamed or swollen, and pressure equalization in the ears may be impaired.

WHAT TO DO: Very often, you can expect that frequent swallowing and yawning (which you can force) will help to combat the pressure disturbance and discomfort. Gum chewing also can be helpful. If discomfort or hearing difficulty continues for several hours after a flight, it may be necessary to consult a physician, but this is rarely the case.

Helpful, too, as a preventive measure: use of decongestant nose drops or inhalant shortly before or during descent. An oral antihistamine drug taken an hour before boarding may be prophylactic.

Babies often are susceptible to barotitis media, and it is advisable to give a pacifier, formula, or water during descent so swallowing will help keep the eustachian tubes open.

Sinus Pain

If you have a *sinus condition*, you may sometimes experience pain over the affected sinus or sinuses because of obstruction that prevents ready pressure equalization inside and outside the sinus or sinuses. The problem is called *barosinusitis*.

WHAT TO DO: Treatment and prevention of barosinusitis are the same as for the ear condition of barotitis media. Use of a decongestant nasal spray just before descent is likely to be especially helpful.

Allergies

An allergy is an unusual reaction in one person to a substance that is generally harmless for most other people. Foods, drugs, substances in air, pet danders, clothing, jewelry, cosmetics, even temperature can be *allergens* (substances provoking allergic reactions) for those sensitive to them. Well over 20 million Americans have one form of allergy or another.

Usually medical help will be needed to determine the cause of an allergy and provide treatment for it. But there are situations in which you may be able to detect the culprit yourself and avoid it or take effective measures against it. If you have a known severe allergy, you may need to be prepared to treat it as an emergency by carrying appropriate medications with you.

Hay Fever

Capable of producing clogged sinuses, nasal stuffiness, sneezing, eye tearing, and general misery, hay fever can be caused by the pollen dust of trees, plants, and weeds.

Drugstores, of course, are well stocked with remedies. They include antihistamines such as Chlor-Trimeton Allergy Tablets and Syrup, Decapryn Syrup, Dimetane Elixir and Tablets. Antihistamines, in fact, are a mainstay of hay fever treatment, often offering rapid, temporary relief. Serious side effects from the drugs are rare, but a common complaint is drowsiness, which can be dangerous if you drive or work near machinery. Some people develop tolerance to the drowsiness after a time, and there can be some degree of difference in the drowsiness effect of various antihistamines for different individuals. It is also true that one antihistamine, satisfactory for a time, loses its symptom-relieving qualities, and you may have to search for another that may be satisfactory.

Oral decongestants such as D-Feda Syrup, Novafed Liquid, or Sudafed Tablets are often used. They temporarily reduce swelling of the nasal mucous membrane, overcoming clogged nose. Although there are topical products—sprays and drops —they are generally best avoided for a problem like hay fever for which many weeks of treatment are needed. Oral decongestants are not as fast-acting but they have less addictive potential.

Some hay fever sufferers use antihistamine-decongestant combinations such as Allerest Allergy Tablets, R.M. Allergy Relief Medicine Tablets, Chlor-Trimeton Decongestant Tablets, Fedahist Tablets, Fedahist Syrup, Novafed A Liquid, Novahistine Elixir. Combinations are convenient. But with a fixed combination, you get dosages that may or may not be precisely right for you. And it is always best to use minimum effective dosages, as few times a day and for as short a period of time as possible.

If nonprescription preparations are not helpful, a physician may prescribe a more potent prescription product or use desensitization treatment aimed at building up tolerance through a series of injections.

Even if you do find a satisfactory nonprescription product, you should seek medical help at the first indication of a complication. Such complications include pain or popping sounds in the ear; pain above the teeth, in the cheeks, above the eyes, or on the side of the nose, indicating possible sinus infection;

persistent coughing, wheezing, and difficult breathing, indicating possible asthma.

Perennial or Year-Round Allergic Rhinitis

This is similar to hay fever but may extend through much or all of the year rather than occur on a seasonal basis. Medical help is often needed for such allergy. But a recent study with more than 800 patients suggests that home humidification during the winter often can be surprisingly helpful.

Over a three-year period, the study found that with humidification such previous winter-long symptoms as dryness of the nose, throat, and chest were markedly reduced; breathing improved, permitting more restful sleep; the need to clear breathing passages of mucus in the morning decreased. Most of the patients, too, were free of respiratory infections during the winter for the first time in years. If you have a hot-air heating system, humidification can be achieved with a device that attaches to the system or furnace; if you have other types of heating, room humidifiers can be used.

Mold Allergy

Sensitivity to molds can sometimes produce nasal congestion, stuffiness, and other symptoms. Several measures are helpful for such sensitivity. Keeping dust accumulation to a minimum and eliminating plants from the home can reduce exposure to molds. A dry, well-ventilated and well-lighted basement also tends to discourage mold growth.

A measure that is often very useful—if it is possible for the family to be away from home for two or three days—is to place a coffee can containing a small amount of formaldehyde in each room of the house. Left in place for 24 hours, the formaldehyde often eliminates molds for as long as six months. After its use, the house must be well aired. Formaldehyde is a dangerous substance; it should not be left in the reach of children.

Skin Allergies

Almost any substance coming into contact with the skin can cause redness, rash, and itching in those sensitive to it. But recent studies at ten major medical centers have identified leading troublemakers.

At the head of the list is nickel sulfate, often used in the making of inexpensive watches, earrings, rings, and bracelets. As many as 11 percent of those who wear such jewelry eventually experience allergic reactions.

Another major item is potassium dichromate, a substance commonly found in tanned leather, to which about 8 percent of the population is sensitive.

Common household antiseptics are also responsible for many allergic reactions. One, thimerosal (Merthiolate), can trigger attacks in 8 to 10 percent of users.

And an ingredient in many hair dyes, p-phenylenediamine, produces itching and other symptoms in 8 percent of users.

The solution to such skin problems is to suspect possible culprits, narrow in on the actual one, and remove it from contact with the skin. Often you can do this for yourself.

Drug Allergies

Although penicillin is the drug best known for causing allergic reactions—sometimes severe and life-threatening anaphylactic shock (see p. 30)—there are sensitivities in some people to other drugs, including tetracycline antibiotics, sulfa compounds, insulin, tranquilizers, and aspirin. If you are taking a drug that is new for you and develop an allergic response, you should call your physician without undue delay to find out if it is likely to be responsible for your allergic symptoms and whether it can be stopped safely and possibly a switch made to another drug.

A note about aspirin: As valuable as it is, aspirin is not well tolerated by about 0.9 percent of the general population. But if you have other allergy problems, your chances of being allergic to aspirin are increased—to 1.4 percent with hay fever or nasal congestion problems, to 3.8 percent with asthma.

Food Allergies

By far the chief offenders among food allergens are cow's milk, chocolate and cola (the kola nut family), corn, eggs, the pea family (chiefly peanut, which is not a nut), citrus fruits, tomato, wheat and other small grains, cinnamon, and artificial food colors.

Cow's milk—as important an allergen among adults as among children—may produce nasal and bronchial congestion, with excessive mucus production. It can also be responsible in some cases for constipation, diarrhea, abdominal pain, and distention.

Chocolate and cola may produce headache and in some cases are important factors in asthma, year-round rhinitis (running nose), and eczema.

Corn sensitivity may produce headache. It also can lead to allergic tension (insomnia, irritability, restlessness) and allergic fatigue (sleepiness, torpor, weakness, vague aching).

Egg may cause almost any allergic manifestation and is most likely to trigger hives and angioedema (giant hives, with sudden temporary appearance of large skin and mucous membrane wheals and intense itching). Egg also may contribute to eczema, asthma, headache, and gastrointestinal upsets.

In the pea family, the peanut is the most common offender. Mature beans and peas are more often problems than are green peas and snap beans. Pea family members can cause headache and may be involved in asthma, hives, and angioedema.

Oranges, lemons, limes, grapefruits, and tangerines may cause eczema and hives and are sometimes factors in canker sores and asthma.

Tomato is a relatively common cause of eczema, hives, and canker sores; it seldom induces headaches but may cause asthma.

Of the small grains—wheat, rice, barley, oats, wild rice, millet, and rye—wheat is the most allergenic, rye the least. Manifestations of grain allergy include asthma and gastrointestinal disturbances.

Cinnamon is a common cause of hives and headache and an occasional cause of asthma.

Artificial food colors are used in carbonated beverages, breakfast drinks, bubble gum, gelatin desserts, and many medications. The most important allergens among them are the red dye amaranth and the yellow dye tartrazine. Hives and asthma are the most common manifestations.

Other food allergens include pork, beef, onion, garlic, white potato, fish of all kinds, coffee, shrimp, banana, walnut, and pecan. Almost any other food can be allergic for some people.

Foods least likely to be troublesome are chicken, turkey, lamb, rabbit; beet, spinach, cabbage, cauliflower, broccoli, turnip, Brussels sprouts, squash, lettuce, carrot, celery, sweet potato; plum, cherry, apricot, cranberry, blueberry, fig; tea, olives, tapioca, sugar.

If one food is suspected, it can be removed from the diet for three weeks; if symptoms subside, the food can be reintroduced to see if symptoms return. If several foods are suspected, all can be removed for three weeks. One is then returned, and later, at two-day intervals, the others are reintroduced to determine which one or several may be the troublemakers.

Cold Urticaria

In this little known but not rare allergy, the victim breaks out with hives, not because of a food, inhalant or chemical, but because of sensitivity to cold. Lips may swell and hives may appear when ice cream is eaten; hands may puff up and generalized hives appear when a cold object is gripped; hives may appear and there may even be loss of consciousness while swimming in cold water.

For this allergy, your physician can prescribe an antihistamine drug, cyproheptadine, which has been reported to produce good results.

Insect Allergies

The stings of bees, wasps, hornets, and yellow jackets can produce allergic reactions and sometimes dangerous anaphylactic shock. (See INSECT BITES AND STINGS.)

Amebic Dysentery (See WORM-INDUCED DISEASES)

Angioneurotic Edema (See HIVES AND GIANT HIVES)

Appendicitis

Appendicitis can cause serious problems if neglected. It is no less true that unjustified fear (that it may be present when, in fact, it is not) is also responsible for much needless anxiety.

Yet it is possible for you to determine with reasonable accuracy, when you may and may not have appendicitis. Moreover, if you should find yourself in a situation where you are far from medical aid and must take steps not only to diagnose your own or someone else's appendicitis but also to keep it under good control until expert help is available, it's eminently possible for you to do so.

Basic Guidelines

If you look at your own abdomen in a mirror, you'll note that the navel (umbilicus) is essentially in the center. Now draw an imaginary line vertically down the middle of the body from the rib cage through the navel to the crotch. Draw another imaginary line horizontally across the navel. Now you've divided the abdomen into the four quadrants that physicians work by.

Above the imaginary horizontal line are right and left upper quadrants (referring to the patient's right and left); below, right and left lower quadrants.

It is the right lower quadrant that is of interest for appendicitis. It's in this quadrant that the small intestine joins with and opens into the beginning of the large intestine or colon.

The joining is queer—reminiscent of a T-junction on a road. The left part of the T is a dead end. The intestinal contents bypass it, moving to the right. The dead end—a sac called the *cecum* (from the Latin for "blind")—has no known function in man, although in rabbits and other herbivorous animals it is large and serves as a kind of fermentation vat.

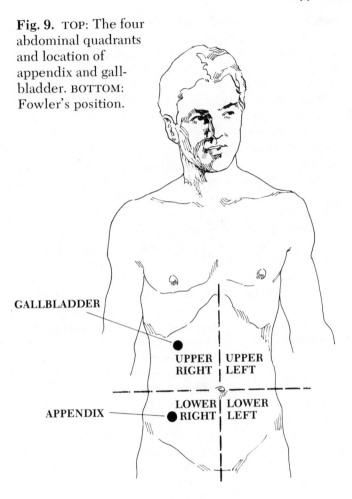

Fig. 9. TOP: The four abdominal quadrants and location of appendix and gall-bladder. BOTTOM: Fowler's position.

GALLBLADDER

UPPER RIGHT | UPPER LEFT

APPENDIX

LOWER RIGHT | LOWER LEFT

FOWLER'S POSITION

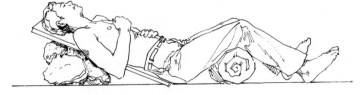

In man the cecum is small, and hanging from it is what is called the *vermiform appendix, vermiform* meaning worm-like, and *appendix* meaning something added on to a main structure. The appendix resembles a fairly fat worm. Commonly, it's about as long as a man's index finger, though it can reach a 10-inch length. Although it has no definitely established purpose, there it hangs, nourished by an artery and drained by a vein system.

In *appendicitis* (the ending "itis" means inflamed or infected), the appendix is inflamed. That happens when the opening between the cecum and appendix is blocked. The blockage can occur when a *fecalith* (a stone made of feces) gets in and fills the entrance to the appendix. Sometimes, a small fruit pit can do the same thing.

But neither fecalith nor pit is essential. An infection present in the area—or even a generalized infection—can cause tissue swelling enough to block the opening.

With the blockage, secretions that ordinarily empty from the appendix into the large intestine accumulate, and the whole appendix begins to swell. And it is at this point that symptoms first occur—but they are not localized to the appendix and can be foolers unless you understand, readily enough, how they develop and what is going on to account for them.

If you were to insert a needle through your abdomen, you would feel pain in the skin and underskin tissues—and pain, too, as the needle penetrates the peritoneum, a thin membrane that looks much like Saran Wrap and lines the abdominal cavity and also covers almost every organ within the abdomen individually. But the intestines and other abdominal organs are insensitive to pain. An anesthetic such as Novocain must be injected into the skin down to the peritoneum in order to cut through without causing pain. But you can then cut into the intestine without using anesthesia and this will not cause any pain.

The appendix does have a nerve supply which it shares with other areas. And as appendicitis begins to develop, although there is as yet no pain in the right lower quadrant of the abdomen where the appendix is, the distention of the blocked organ is signaled through the nerves, and at this point the first symptom occurs: nausea or "upset stomach" which may progress to vomiting.

As the appendix swells still more, another symptom appears: a typical pain around the navel (medically known as *periumbilical pain*), not even close to where the appendix lies. Here, in this pain, we have an interesting phenomenon —referred pain. With the appendix increasingly diseased, messages are transmitted by nerves to the spinal cord and brain, and since those nerves also supply other areas, the brain interprets the pain as coming from the periumbilical area.

But more is to come. With still further swelling of the appendix, veins carrying blood from it become blocked off, blood stagnates within the appendix, and bacteria, no longer carried away in the blood, multiply.

Now the infection intensifies and affects the wall of the appendix. And as the wall becomes infected, it inflames the peritoneum of the abdominal wall which it touches. Because the peritoneum is pain-sensitive, symptoms change.

Now, for the first time, comes severe pain in the right lower quadrant. The previous periumbilical pain has migrated.

Moreover, now, if you press on the right lower quadrant, the area is tender. And, in fact, because inflammation of the peritoneum can cause spasm, or involuntary contraction, of abdominal muscles in the area, when you press on the right lower quadrant you can feel that is no longer soft, as it normally should be, but now is firm, even rigid.

THE 1, 2, 3 PROGRESSION:

So now we have a 1, 2, 3 progression of symptoms which can point to acute appendicitis:

1. Nausea or upset stomach which may go to to vomiting
2. Periumbilical pain
3. Right lower quadrant pain and tenderness

As with any disease, there can be variations in symptoms. Those I have described, however, are most typical.

What to Do

When the 1, 2, 3 progression of symptoms points to appendicitis as being likely, medical help should be sought without delay. (I will deal later with what you can do when medical help is not available.)

The physician who performs an examination for acute appendicitis will—or should—insert a gloved finger into the rectum. When he presses, interiorly, at the point of the inflammation of the peritoneum, it will be tender.

He will do both a simple blood test and a urinalysis. Both are important.

The blood test checks for the number of white blood cells. With any infection, white cells, part of the body defense system, increase in numbers in order to try to kill the infectious organisms. So their increased numbers indicate infection.

The urinalysis checks for any blood or pus in the urine. The reason for a urinalysis: Very close to the appendix runs the ureter, the tube from the right kidney carrying urine to the bladder. If there should be a stone or infection in the urinary system, it could produce symptoms similar to those of appendicitis.

Once the symptoms, plus the tests mentioned, confirm the probability of appendicitis, surgery is indicated. An *appendectomy* today is usually a relatively simple procedure. The appendix can be reached through a 2- or 3-inch abdominal incision. The base of the appendix, where it originates at the cecum, is tied off, and the organ is then removed.

The complete operation, from opening the abdomen to suturing it closed again at the end, carried out under general or spinal anesthesia, can take half an hour or less. Commonly, the patient is up next day, eating a normal diet within a few days, home in 5 to 7 days, with the wound completely healed in 7 to 10 days.

After an appendectomy, the surgeon should not hesitate to tell what he found—even if the appendix turned out to be normal, not diseased.

I must emphasize that in order to try to preclude the risk of having an appendix perforate, leading to peritonitis, surgery is rightly undertaken when there is high probability of appendicitis, but not necessarily complete certainty. It is almost inevitable, therefore, that a busy, skilled surgeon finds, upon operation, that about 15 percent of appendices are normal.

But if the appendix proved to be normal, what accounted for the symptoms? Did he look around in the abdomen to see if there might have been, in the case of a woman, an ovarian cyst or inflamed tube or, in the case of either sex, a stone in the urinary tract that caused the symptoms? There are other diseases—for example, *ileitis*, an inflammation of the lower portion of the small intestine—which may mimic appendicitis.

As a patient, you have the right to know, and to ask the surgeon: was the appendix normal or abnormal? You have the right to know what the pathologist's report (after microscopic examination of the removed tissue) reveals—and, if the appendix was normal, whether the surgeon looked around to see what else might be wrong, and what he found, and what if anything he did. This is extremely important to you if abdominal pain should recur at a later date.

WHAT CAN YOU DO IF YOU'RE ALONE WITH APPENDICITIS: Such a situation could develop, for example, if you're "away from civilization" on a camping, hunting or fishing trip, or on a small boat.

If you're within relatively easy reach of a decent size hospital with an experienced surgeon available, there is no great problem. You can make your own likely diagnosis, know an operation is needed, and get there and have it. If you can be transported there by helicopter, all the better. Obviously, you should not ride horseback for several days to get there; increased activity can cause an inflamed appendix to burst.

If getting medical help quickly is not possible and someone else is the patient, should you try heroic lay surgery? *No. That is dangerous—and unnecessary.*

Wide publicity was given during World War II to a medical corpsman on a submarine who fashioned tools and removed an appendix as the sub lay on the ocean bottom. On a later occasion, a similar appendectomy was performed by a pharmacist's mate on a submarine under attack.

These made good stories and an exciting motion picture. But the Armed Forces not long afterward issued orders that medical corpsmen were not to perform appendectomies under any circumstances; instead the sailor or soldier was to receive intravenous fluids and penicillin for as long as necessary until he could be transferred to a hospital. Apparently, it was realized that such amateur surgery was more dangerous than attempting to control the infection and prevent peritonitis by use of antibiotics.

If you should ever be faced with acute appendicitis where medical help is not available, first, put yourself—and your appendix—at rest. This means lying still in what is known as *Fowler's position* (after Dr. George Fowler, the New York surgeon who discovered its value at the turn of the century). It's a semisitting position, with your back up at least 45 degrees from horizontal and with a blanket roll under the knees to avoid stretching of abdominal muscles. Take no cathartic or enema, and eat or drink nothing.

With Fowler's position, you help to assure that, should the appendix perforate, pus will settle by gravity into the lowest part of the abdomen, and there will be a better chance for an abscess to form and wall off the infection so that it does not spread throughout the abdomen.

Take an antibiotic. Anyone today going off to an isolated (or developing) area should always carry antibiotics prescribed by a physician, with the proper dosage specified by the physician for any infection, including appendicitis, that may develop.

Take the antibiotic by mouth with the minimal amount of water needed for swallowing. Too much fluid may increase nausea and induce vomiting, preventing drug absorption.

The antibiotic will diminish or eliminate the infection, helping even if peritonitis has set in.

Should your mouth feel dry and your urine diminish, it is important to keep your circulating fluids up. So, once nausea has passed, sip small amounts of water throughout the day. Or you can sip tea with lemon and a little sugar. A little clear broth with some salt in it also will be helpful. Do not drink full-strength fruit juices or coffee, which may stimulate bowel contraction.

If fever should develop, take aspirin or acetaminophen, two tablets every three hours or so.

There has been much discussion about whether or not an ice or cold pack on the right lower quadrant has any value in controlling appendicitis. Theoretically, cold could diminish the spread of inflammation. The general feeling, however, has been and still largely is that the cold does not get into the abdomen—although some recent animal studies suggest that it does, in fact, do so. Be that as it may, a cold pack over the area is helpful in diminishing discomfort and, in so doing, will enable you, and therefore your intestine, to rest more comfortably.

Should pain still be severe and you have along a narcotic such as codeine or a sleeping pill such as pentobarbital (Nembutal), take it in the doses your physician suggested when he prescribed.

None of this, of course, is a substitute for surgery. But with these measures you almost certainly can keep matters under control safely until expert surgery is available.

Arm Pain, Coldness, Numbness, Tingling, Blanching, Swelling

When sudden coldness, tingling, and numbness develop in an arm and are followed by severe pain, blanching or mottling of the skin with blue patches, the cause may be blockage of an artery in the arm, requiring medical help. (See ARTERY BLOCKAGE, ARM OR LEG.)

Sudden pain in an arm may indicate a bone break. (See FRACTURES.)

Sudden swelling of an arm, with increased warmth of the skin, may indicate infection but also may be due to a vein clot. (See VENOUS THROMBOSIS.)

Artery Blockage, Arm or Leg

When an arm or leg artery is suddenly blocked, or occluded, the first symptoms may be coldness, numbness, and tingling.

Soon, severe pain and blanching or mottling of the skin with blue patches may follow.

The blockage can be the result of development of a blood clot in an artery already narrowed by deposits on its wall caused by the disease atherosclerosis. Another possibility is that a clot (embolus) originating elsewhere is carried to the arm or leg artery in the bloodstream and becomes lodged there.

WHAT TO DO: A doctor should be seen as quickly as possible. Immediate medical treatment may include use of anti-clotting drugs (anticoagulants) along with other measures such as injections of procaine and papaverine, and improvement may begin within a few hours. If improvement does not occur, the clot may be removed, without further delay, through an incision in the artery.

Athlete's Foot

Also known as *tinea pedis* and *ringworm of the foot,* athlete's foot is a common, sometimes resistant nuisance. At its peak, with malodorous, soggy, whitish, itching lesions between the toes, it can be severely annoying.

Recently, new insights into the nature of the condition and its treatment have been obtained.

Athlete's foot starts out, as long known, as an infection caused by a fungus (a microscopic plant growth) that is commonly found in locker rooms, public showers, and swimming pool walkways and thrives on dead cells of the skin between the toes.

Early on, a mild fungus-killing ointment or powder obtainable at your drugstore may be effective, especially when combined with good foot care, including gentle removal of scales, bathing, and scrupulous drying. Use of absorbent cotton or wool socks, rather than synthetics, may be helpful.

But recent studies indicate that while athlete's foot starts out as a fungal infection, when it becomes really troublesome —with odor, itching, and other annoying symptoms—the fungi no longer are active and may not even be present. Bacteria are the culprits.

The scenario, it seems, goes like this: First, the fungi, multiplying between the toes, produce skin scaling. Then, at some point, excessive moisture is introduced—because of exercise, hot weather, tight shoes, or other factors. The moisture provides an ideal environment for bacteria, which multiply rapidly and may even drive out the fungi, producing the acute symptoms.

At that point, more effective than an antifungal preparation may be one capable of doing two things: combating bacteria and assuring drying.

Such a preparation, recent research suggests, is a solution of 30 percent aluminum chloride ($AlCl_36H_2O$), which your druggist can prepare relatively inexpensively. In clinical trials, the solution, applied twice a day with a cotton-tipped applicator, usually relieved itching and ended malodor within 48 to 72 hours. The solution can be applied until complete clearance has occurred. Thereafter, it may be needed only once a day in very hot, humid weather. *Caution:* The solution can be irritating and should not be used in the presence of fissures—narrow, deep slits—which allow it to penetrate too deeply. Ointments and powders should then be used.

If, despite appropriate home care, athlete's foot persists, do see a physician, who may prescribe antifungal antibiotic and other measures.

Back Pain

Pain low in the back can sometimes stem from problems not related to the back. For example, severe, increasing back pain, just under the ribs and on one side only, may be due to kidney disease (see KIDNEY STONE).

But far more common is the kind of low back pain that may be triggered by a fall, blow, heavy lifting, shoveling snow, changing a tire, other strenuous exertion, and even, on occasion, by something as simple as bending over to tie a shoelace or sitting for a prolonged period at a meeting. Whatever the trigger, the pain is usually severe, with difficulty in walking and standing.

WHAT TO DO: Acute back pain often can be relieved by home measures if they are used properly.

The first thing to do is to take two aspirins (or acetaminophen, if aspirin doesn't set well with you) and, if possible, lie down. As soon thereafter as you can, get into bed. If the mattress is firm, so much the better. If there is a bed board under the mattress, still better.

Start at once to apply heat, using a heating pad within a Turkish towel. Apply for half an hour, then shift position to avoid stiffness.

If heat doesn't help, try cold—gently rubbing the painful area with crushed ice or ice cubes in a pillowcase.

Either heat or cold—one or the other may work better for you—helps combat muscle spasm, which is involuntary contraction of muscles, a body defense mechanism to splint a painful area. The trouble, though, is that spasm, after a time, produces pain, the increased pain produces more spasm, and a vicious cycle is set up.

Have someone give you a rubdown with a counterirritant, any commercially available one.

Use all of the foregoing measures rather than relying on just one.

And repeat them. For most people, two aspirin tablets every three to four hours as needed, if taken for no more than one or two days, often are helpful and not dangerous. Prolonged intake of aspirin, however, can cause complications such as gastrointestinal bleeding for some people. Repeat the heat or cold applications, too. If you are using heat and can make it to a bathtub, a warm bath (much better than a shower) for 30 minutes four or even more times a day is in order. So, too, the massage—gentle, easy rubbing—several times a day.

After a day or two, perhaps overnight, you may find the pain easing. Gently and slowly move your arms and legs, and arch and curve the back to keep from getting stiff. Continue the aspirin, hot or cold applications, massage, and stretching motions.

The measures I have been discussing are for a very severe episode. Many acute episodes produce much less severe pain and do not necessarily require bed rest. If you experience a milder episode, reduce all physical activities while remaining out of bed, and use aspirin, hot or cold applications, counterirritant, and massage.

If the pain of a severe episode is undiminished after a day or so, you should consult your physician. You may need more potent pain-relieving medication or other measures.

PREVENTION: Once an acute attack is over, you can take steps to prevent recurrences.

A major factor in setting the stage for back pain attacks is weakness not so much of back muscles but of abdominal muscles. Unless special attention is paid to the latter, they are rarely exercised and commonly are flabby. Both the abdominal and back muscles combine to support the back. When the abdominals are weak, the burden on the back muscles is increased, and they tend to fatigue more easily and to become more readily subject to injury.

Special exercises to strengthen the abdominal muscles can do much to prevent recurrences and are often valuable even when a spinal disk problem may be involved (see the following section). Many YMCAs now are offering exercise programs for backache victims. A valuable source of information about backaches of all types, which also provides a graduated exercise program, is a book, *Freedom from Backaches,* by Lawrence W. Friedmann, M.D., of the State University of New York School of Medicine, Stony Brook, and Lawrence Galton (Simon & Schuster).

Back Pain with Leg Pain (Sciatica)

The sciatic nerve, one of the longest in the body, extends from the base of the spine down the thigh and has branches throughout the lower leg and foot. In sciatica, the nerve is inflamed, producing pain that may begin in the buttock and extend down the back of the thigh and leg to the ankle.

Sciatica may occur with low back pain or independently. It can result from *osteoarthritis* (wear-and-tear arthritis) of the spine. Sometimes a damaged spinal disk may be responsible, setting up the inflammation by pressing on the sciatic nerve at a point where it originates in the spine. Sometimes, sciatica much like that from a disk problem develops when a muscle in spasm puts pressure on the nerve (physicians often refer to this as *pseudodisk syndrome*).

In most cases, sciatica responds to measures very much like those for back pain: aspirin or acetaminophen, use of a firm mattress, local heat or cold applications.

If the leg pain persists, a physician can help. Surgery is sometimes necessary, but avoid it if you possibly can. Although a disk operation often dramatically relieves pain, in many cases the symptoms persist.

Bites, Animal (See also INSECT AND OTHER BUG BITES AND STINGS)

WHAT TO DO: The first thing to do for an animal bite is to immediately wash the wound with water to remove the animal's saliva. Then spend five minutes thoroughly cleansing the wound with soap and water. Rinse thoroughly. Cover with a dressing unless the bite has left a cut or puncture wound, in which case see CUTS or WOUNDS, PUNCTURE.

What of possible infection, rabies, and need for medical attention?

Any animal bite—from dog, cat, rat, bat, raccoon, or other wild animal—may possibly carry rabies and may need medical attention without delay. If the bite is from a pet dog or cat or from someone else's pet, and the animal's immunizations are current and you can rely on the owner to observe the animal for the next two weeks to make certain it shows no indications of rabies, then you may not need to see a physician immediately in terms of possible rabies. You should, however, report the incident to him. If the animal does develop indications of rabies, immediate medical attention is urgent.

There are three types of indications of rabies in an animal. The first two may be classified as either "furious" or "dumb." Furious rabies in a dog is characterized by agitation, viciousness, then paralysis and death; dumb rabies in a dog is manifested mainly by paralytic symptoms. More often rabid animals show a third type of behavioral change which is more subtle, such as lack of normal fear of humans or activity by day in such animals as bats, skunks, and foxes which ordinarily are active by night.

If the animal is strange and not available for observation, see a physician immediately after thoroughly cleansing the wound. Rabies can be deadly. Fortunately, thorough cleansing is of great value in prevention. Fortunately, too, immunization of dogs has greatly decreased rabies transmission. Still, the possible need for antirabies injections may have to be considered, especially if there has been a severe wound of the head or face. Human symptoms of rabies can appear anywhere from ten days to two years after a bite, with the average being about two months—but the incubation is shorter when the wound is on the head or even the neck rather than on an arm or leg, since it is related to distance from wound to brain.

Infection other than with rabies virus is possible but not common after an animal bite. Tetanus is one possibility, and if you have not had a tetanus shot for a long time, your physician may want to administer one; you can check on this by phone.

As with any other puncture wound, other infection may possibly develop. If it does, it will take at least 24 hours to do so. Watch for fever, pus, severe swelling, and redness; if these appear, have a physician examine the wound and perhaps prescribe an antibiotic.

Bites, Human

Because the human mouth contains many bacteria, there is some possibility that a human bite that breaks the skin may become infected.

There is, in fact, no infection worse than that which may come from a human bite. If, by accident or purposefully, you strike someone in the teeth and there is an opening through your skin, act immediately.

WHAT TO DO: Cleanse thoroughly, rinsing away saliva, then washing vigorously with soap and water. Cover the wound with gauze, but do not close off all air by covering with tape. Check with a physician about need for further treatment.

Bites, Snake

Two principal types of poisonous snakes—coral snakes and pit vipers—are found in the United States.

Coral snakes occur from North Carolina through Florida, westward to Texas, and up the Mississippi Valley to Indiana.

The pit viper family includes rattlesnakes, copperheads, and cottonmouth moccasins and may be found in many areas of the country.

Pit vipers have a characteristic indented pit between eye and nostril on each side of the head. Their venom affects the blood circulation system.

The coral snake, a variety of cobra, is small, has red, yellow and black rings around the body, and black nose. Its toxic venom affects the nervous system.

WHAT TO DO: First, have the victim lie down quietly to slow blood circulation and spread of the venom.

If the bite is on an arm or leg, apply a tourniquet between the bite and the rest of body, using anything—belt, tie, rope, or strip of cloth—you can wrap and firmly tie around, but not too tightly. If properly tied, there should be some oozing from the wound and you should be able to slip your index finger under the band.

Stop a moment and consider: Is the bite poisonous?

A bite by a rattlesnake, copperhead, or moccasin will immediately produce stinging pain, rapid swelling, and skin discoloration. Later may come weakness, rapid pulse, nausea and vomiting, shortness of breath, vision dimness, and shock.

A coral snake bite may produce only slight burning pain and mild local swelling at the wound, but other symptoms will appear in a few minutes, including blurring of vision, drooping of eyelids, slurring of speech, drowsiness, sweating, increased salivation, breathing difficulty, and nausea.

If no physician is available and you believe the bite to be poisonous, sterilize a knife blade or razor blade with a flame. Make cuts through the skin at each fang mark—and also just a little lower than the fang marks where the venom is most likely to have been deposited. Make the cuts through the skin only and in the long axis of the limb. If you go deeper than the skin, you may sever muscles and nerves.

Then suck out the venom. If you have a snakebite kit with a suction cup, use the cup. Otherwise, use your mouth. Snake venom is not a stomach poison and you can spit it out and rinse it from your mouth. Suction is very valuable; if done quickly and properly, it can remove most of the venom. Keep up the suction for 30 to 60 minutes. If swelling begins to extend up to the tourniquet, leave that one in place but apply another a few inches above.

Thoroughly wash the wound with soap and water, blot dry, and apply sterile or clean dressing and bandage.

Get medical help as soon as you can for possible use of antivenin. If the snake has been killed, take it with you for identification.

Give no alcohol. If the victim is not nauseous and can swallow without difficulty, give sips of fluid.

If necessary, use artificial respiration (p. 49). Also, if necessary, treat for shock (p. 28).

Even if a bite has been by a nonpoisonous snake, check with a physician about possible need for antibiotic treatment and tetanus prevention.

Bladder Infection (See URINARY TRACT INFECTIONS)

Bleeding

Some bleeding—from capillaries, the tiniest of blood vessels—amounts to only an oozing of blood.

Bleeding from a vein—identifiable because the blood is dark red—is usually slow and even.

Bleeding from an artery—with the blood bright red in color —may be profuse. With each heartbeat, the blood may spurt from the wound. Arterial bleeding is much less common than capillary or vein bleeding because larger arteries are well protected within body tissues and not often subject to injury.

What to Do

You can almost always control bleeding, even when it is heavy, by proceeding calmly with certain definite steps.

APPLY PRESSURE: This works for minor bleeding and more often than not for even severe bleeding. And it is a preferable method because it prevents blood loss without interfering with normal circulation.

Apply a sterile gauze pad over the wound. If a pad is not immediately available, use a clean handkerchief, clean cloth, even an item of clothing, especially if the bleeding is heavy. When bleeding is profuse, rather than delay, use even your bare hand and worry about infection later.

Press the pad—or bare hand—directly over the wound. Most bleeding can be controlled by pressure. Once you have it under some control, apply cloth material if you have used your hand. A thick pad helps to encourage clotting of blood. A feminine sanitary pad is very effective. If you have already used gauze or cloth, apply additional layers. Then apply a tight roller bandage or cravat to maintain pressure. If you have nothing else available, use cloth strips or neckties.

Do *not* remove the bandage. If blood saturates it, add more layers of gauze or cloth and tighten the whole dressing over the wound. Take care, of course, not to wrap the pressure dressing so tightly that circulation is cut off.

Note: Clotting of blood is the body's means for controlling hemorrhage, but clotting may take as long as *three to ten minutes* so maintain direct pressure *for at least that long.*

ELEVATE: If no bones are broken, it helps to raise the bleeding part higher than the rest of the body. Because of the force of gravity, elevation tends to reduce blood flow to the injured site.

INDIRECT PRESSURE (PRESSURE POINTS): If direct pressure

on the wound fails to stop the flow, indirect pressure—also called pressure point control—can be added. It consists of applying pressure to the artery supplying blood to the injury site. Remember: always compress the artery at a point between the heart and the bleeding site.

There are several points where that can be done, compressing the artery against a bone with your fingers or hand to check blood flow.

For an arm wound: Use the *brachial artery*. You'll find the pressure point on the inside of the arm, about halfway between the elbow and armpit, in the groove between the biceps and triceps (the front and back muscles of the upper arm). Place your thumb on the outside of the arm and press your fingers on the inside of the arm toward the thumb, using not the fingertips but the flat inside surfaces of the fingers.

For a leg wound: Use the *femoral artery*. The pressure point is on the inner thigh at the crease of the groin. With the heel of your hand there, press against the bone.

For a scalp wound: Use the *temporal artery*. The pressure point is at the side of the head just in front of the ear. You may have to press on both sides of the head to gain control, as the circulation extends across the head.

For a cheek wound: Use the *facial artery*. The pressure point is midway along the jaw, between ear and chin.

For head and neck bleeding: Use the *carotid artery*. The pressure point is on the side of the neck below the jaw, just before but not over the windpipe.

For chest, shoulder, or armpit bleeding: Use the *subclavian artery*. Press with your thumb in the groove behind the collarbone.

Note: Even the most severe hemorrhage will likely be controlled by a combination of pressure dressing at the wound site and indirect pressure at the pressure point for the supplying artery—*if the pressure is maintained long enough to permit clotting.*

ONLY AS A LAST RESORT: A TOURNIQUET: Tourniquets are rarely needed. They are used much too often, and they can be dangerous.

If you use a tourniquet, it should be only as a last resort to

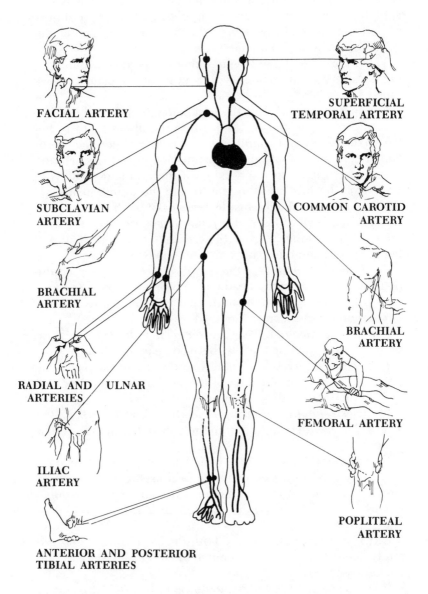

FACIAL ARTERY

SUPERFICIAL TEMPORAL ARTERY

SUBCLAVIAN ARTERY

COMMON CAROTID ARTERY

BRACHIAL ARTERY

BRACHIAL ARTERY

RADIAL AND ULNAR ARTERIES

FEMORAL ARTERY

ILIAC ARTERY

POPLITEAL ARTERY

ANTERIOR AND POSTERIOR TIBIAL ARTERIES

Fig. 10. Pressure points for control of bleeding.

save life, with an understanding that what is involved may be the sacrifice of a limb to save life. When a tourniquet is applied, circulation to all points below it is cut off. If the tourniquet is left on for an extended period, gangrene (tissue death) may follow and amputation may be required.

If a tourniquet must be used, proceed thus:

1. Use a tourniquet at least two inches wide. If a commercial tourniquet is not available, use a triangular bandage, towel, or handkerchief folded several times.
2. Place the tourniquet above and close to the edge of the wound. To be effective, as already noted, it must be between the wound and the heart.
3. Wrap the tourniquet tightly around the limb and secure it with a single knot.
4. Place a short, strong stick or similar object on the knot and tie two more knots on top.

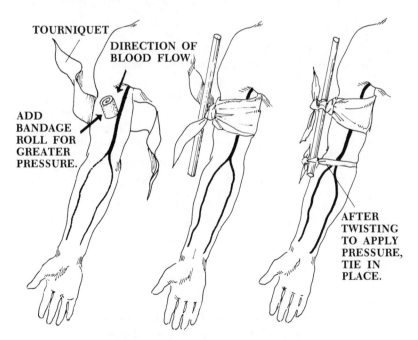

Fig. 11. Applying a tourniquet.

5. Twist the stick to tighten the tourniquet only enough to stop the bleeding. Then secure the stick with a strip of cloth or other material.
6. Once applied, do not loosen the tourniquet unless instructed to do so by a physician.
7. Immediately after applying the tourniquet, note the time and attach the note in a prominent location on the victim's clothes.
8. Treat for shock (see p. 28).

Bleeding from the Nose

Nosebleeds are common. They can be caused by injury, picking the nose, excessive sneezing or coughing, or exposure to very dry air. High blood pressure may be responsible. Some people, too, have blood vessels in the nose that are delicate and easily ruptured.

Generally, nosebleeds are more nuisances than serious matters, last for only a few minutes, and are easy to control. A slight nosebleed, in fact, usually stops by itself.

If, however, bleeding continues or is severe, a few simple measures usually can be counted on to help.

WHAT TO DO: Sit upright in a chair and stay as quiet as possible. Do not tilt your head backward: keep it in normal position. By sitting up quietly, rather than lying down, you allow the blood to run out of the front of the nose rather than down the back of the throat. The latter could conceal the fact that bleeding is continuing; it also opens up some possibility that the blood may get into the lungs. Moreover, sitting up tends to lower pressure of blood in the veins, and if the bleeding from the nose is from a vein, which is most common, the vein has a better chance to collapse.

Apply pressure at the bleeding site by pressing the outside of the nostril toward the midline of the nose against the bony cartilage there. This is the equivalent of applying pressure to a bleeding site elsewhere in the body. And here, as elsewhere, if you maintain the pressure for at least three minutes

—preferably a little longer to be safe—the blood can clot and bleeding stop.

Applying cold compresses or ice packs to the nose and face —especially above the nose or across the bridge of the nose —may help control the bleeding.

In the rare event that the bleeding persists more than 10 or 15 minutes or is obviously bright red and profuse (thus indicating that it is coming from an artery), maintain pressure on the nostril and do not let go until you can reach a physician or get to a hospital emergency room.

Note: If you have persistently recurring nosebleeds, they warrant medical attention to determine the underlying cause. Previously undiscovered high blood pressure may be involved or possibly some fault in the blood's clotting mechanism. These problems, or any others that may account for repeated nosebleeds, should and can be treated.

Bleeding, Internal

Bleeding within the body—without a break in the skin— may make itself known through vomiting or coughing up blood (which may have a "coffee grounds" rather than red appearance), blood in the stool (which also may not be red but instead may give the stool a black or tarry appearance), or hemorrhaging from a body opening such as mouth, ears, or nose.

But internal bleeding may also develop without visible blood indications, although there will usually be other guides to its presence.

WHEN TO SUSPECT INTERNAL HEMORRHAGE WITHOUT VISIBLE BLEEDING: This type of hemorrhage usually occurs as the result of a crushing or blunt injury to the body—a violent blow which may damage internal organs or blood vessels or both.

After such injury, look for indications of shock, which is a potentially dangerous disruption of blood circulation (see also SHOCK, p. 28).

In the early stages of shock:

1. The skin is pale and may be moist and cool.
2. Weakness is present.
3. The pulse is usually rapid (over 100), and often it may be too weak to be felt at the wrist but may be detected at the carotid artery at the side of the neck.
4. The breathing rate is usually increased and may be irregular.
5. There may be vomiting or retching.
6. Thirst may be severe.
7. There may be restlessness and thrashing about.

Such shock-producing internal bleeding requires medical attention as soon as possible.

WHAT TO DO: Place the victim flat on his back. *Exception:* If he has difficulty breathing, pillow up his head and shoulders. Also elevate his legs; this will return blood from the lower extremities to the heart and brain where its lack is causing the shock state.

Keep him as quiet and reassured as you can.

Try to have him control retching. Turn his head to the side for vomiting.

Give *no* stimulants.

Keep him warm enough with covers to prevent or overcome chilling. Do not use heating pads or other artificial warming methods, as they will increase the circulation rate and blood loss and may burn the skin.

Do not give fluids when the victim is unconscious, vomiting or likely to vomit, or when medical help can be expected within an hour, since surgery to repair the internal injuries may be required.

Get medical help without delay. If necessary to move the victim to a hospital, do so in a flat-on-back or slightly propped position.

Note: Internal bleeding sometimes may not occur immediately after an injury but may develop hours or even days later. This is often due to a tear in the capsule surrounding the spleen. If you have had a severe crushing or blunt injury and only later, even after having had medical attention, experience the indications just noted, waste no time in getting to an emergency room.

Bleeding from the Rectum

The discovery of what appears to be blood in the stool or in the toilet bowl after a bowel movement can be alarming. But alarm is not always justified.

If you are healthy, feel no weakness, have a good strong pulse, and happen to see what looks like bright red blood in a stool, by all means think back a few hours: Did you, for example, have beets for dinner the night before? That could account for what looks like bright red blood. And if the stool looks very dark, did you drink a fair amount of dark red wine, which could account for the color?

A common cause of bright red blood in the toilet bowl is bleeding from a hemorrhoid or pile. That may not constitute an emergency situation but does warrant medical investigation.

The passage of fresh red blood from the rectum typically arises, if not from hemorrhoids, then from sources in the lower intestine. Among possible causes are polyps in the colon, diverticular disease of the colon, ulcerative colitis, and malignancy. Sometimes, however, if bleeding higher up in the gastrointestinal tract—from a bleeding peptic ulcer, for example—is particularly heavy and rapid, there may be red blood in the stool.

Ordinarily, blood from higher up in the GI tract, in passing through the large intestine, becomes black in color, producing black or tarry stools. However, slowly bleeding sites in the large intestine at times can also produce such stools. And black stools may also be due to taking iron or bismuth and eating berries or greens.

Any bleeding from the rectum not due to an obviously harmless source deserves prompt medical attention.

Bleeding—Vomiting Blood

Among the most common causes of vomiting of blood are a peptic ulcer, inflammation of the lining of the stomach called gastritis, and rupture of a blood vessel in the esophagus, the last being almost exclusively limited to people with cirrhosis of the liver.

Vomited blood is not always red in color. When bleeding is slow, stomach juices may have a chance to act on the blood, digesting it somewhat, giving it the appearance of "coffee grounds." Do not be confused by the "coffee grounds" look; it definitely indicates loss of blood.

WHAT TO DO: Medical attention should be sought without delay. The earlier the patient is seen, preferably within a few hours after an episode, the more accurate the diagnosis of where the bleeding is coming from is likely to be.

Note: If you have vomited several times or have retched heavily, a small amount of blood-streaked vomitus may be brought up. This in itself is not dangerous and can be attended to without necessarily rushing to the emergency room as long as other symptoms, notably those indicating shock, do not occur. But note, too, that prolonged, severe vomiting or retching sometimes can cause a tear in the esophagus, leading to severe bleeding and vomiting of blood, requiring immediate hospitalization.

Blister

Generally, if a blister can be protected against breaking, leave it alone. The colorless, watery fluid will be gradually absorbed by deeper layers of skin and the skin will soon return to normal.

If the blister is large or in an area where it is likely to be broken—such as on the foot where it may be opened by shoe rubbing—follow these steps:

1. Gently clean the blister and the area around it with soap and water.

2. Sterilize a needle over a flame and use it to puncture the edge of the blister.
3. Gently press the edges of the blister opposite the point of puncture to force out the fluid slowly.
4. Apply a sterile gauze pad and adhesive.

If a blister has already broken, wash off the area carefully with soap and water, and apply sterile gauze pad and adhesive.

Boils and Carbuncles

A boil is an inflamed, swollen elevation on the skin produced by staphylococcal bacteria. The bacteria, often present on the skin, do no harm until they penetrate, gaining access through hair follicles, sweat glands, or a break in the skin surface resulting from a cut, scratch, or puncture by a pin or tack.

At first the infection causes the skin to become warm, red and tender, at which point it is called a *furuncle*. As part of the body's reaction, the infection is confined by resistance processes to a limited area and pus accumulates at its center. At this point, continued treatment can bring the boil to a "head."

Boils commonly occur on the neck, breast, face, and buttocks but are most painful when situated in skin closely attached to underlying structures (such as on the nose, ear, or fingers).

A carbuncle, which may be produced by the same type of bacteria involved in boils, is more serious than a boil. It is, in effect, a cluster of boils, with inflammation involving not only the skin but deeper tissues, and may be accompanied by fever and a general feeling of illness. Carbuncles occur most often in males and most commonly on the nape of the neck.

WHAT TO DO: Anyone with a carbuncle should see a physician. So should anyone who has a number of boils at one time or suffers from repeated outbreaks. Boils and carbuncles sometimes can be serious matters since organisms from them may enter the blood. This is particularly true of a boil or carbuncle on the nose or upper lip, because in these areas there is an easier access route for the bacteria to get to the brain.

Both boils and carbuncles respond readily to medical treatment, which may include use of a suitable antibiotic, warm (not hot to the touch) soaks, and/or incision and drainage.

Don't ever squeeze a boil. This will break its protective wall and encourage spread of the infection deeper into the skin or other tissues. When a physician opens a boil, he spreads its walls apart to evacuate the enclosed pus, taking care to avoid the danger of bacteria getting into the bloodstream causing blood poisoning (septicemia) and risk of abscess in a vital part of the body.

If you have a small boil that is not on the nose or upper lip, it is usually safe for you to try the following:

1. Wash the boil and surrounding area with soap and water several times a day. Lightly dab on 70 percent alcohol afterward. Cover with an antiseptic gauze pad to prevent irritation.

2. Several times a day, even as often as hourly if possible, apply warm compresses 10 minutes at a time. Make the compresses by soaking an antiseptic gauze pad in warm water containing approximately one full tablespoon of Epsom salt (magnesium sulfate) in a quart of water (940 cc). This helps relieve pain and also stimulates the boil to point, or come to a head, and then drain spontaneously.

3. When the boil does point and discharge, avoid touching any of the pus. Wipe off promptly with a sterile gauze and cover with sterile dressing. Discard the gauze in a wrapping so it cannot contaminate others. Wash your hands thoroughly with soap and water after change of dressing.

If the boil is not better within a few days, see your physician. Do not attempt to deliberately open a boil yourself.

Bone Pain (Osteomyelitis, Bone Infection)

Osteomyelitis is an infection of bone and bone marrow that typically begins with sudden pain in the affected bone. In addition, fever is present, there is tenderness over the bone, and movement is painful and restricted. Later, swelling appears over the bone and often in a nearby joint.

The infection is caused by invading bacteria, which may gain entrance through a compound fracture or other injury, from a nearby infection, or through the blood.

WHAT TO DO: Get medical help without delay. The likelihood of controlling the infection is excellent if treatment with a suitable antibiotic is started with little loss of time. Antibiotic treatment may be needed for as long as 8 to 12 weeks after all signs of swelling and tenderness have disappeared.

Bowel, Irritable (See COLON, IRRITABLE)

Bronchitis

Occurring most often in winter, acute infectious bronchitis, an inflammation of the bronchial tubes, may develop after a common cold or other viral infection of the nose or throat.

There may be the typical symptoms of a cold or other acute respiratory infection: chilliness, slight fever, malaise, sore throat, back and muscle pain, and profuse nasal discharge.

Onset of a cough usually indicates onset of bronchitis. At first the cough is usually dry and nonproductive, but after a few hours or days small amounts of sputum are brought up, and later the sputum becomes more abundant.

In a severe, uncomplicated case of acute bronchitis, fever of up to 102°F may be present for three to five days, after which acute symptoms subside, although cough may continue for two or three weeks. Persistent fever may indicate complicating pneumonia.

WHAT TO DO: Rest is important until fever subsides. Plenty of fluids should be taken. Steam inhalations are helpful. Aspirin or acetaminophen every four to eight hours relieves malaise and reduces fever.

Expectorant drugs may be used. When effective, they loosen secretions in the air passages and increase expectoration. Actually, the proverbial remedy, chicken soup, as long as it has plenty of pepper, garlic and possibly curry powder, can be helpful for the same purpose. Do not let embarrassment cause you to permit secretions to accumulate in the lungs. The cough is nature's way of getting rid of the mucus. Cough it up and spit it out into paper tissue.

For a lingering, nonproductive, irritative cough, either a codeine or other cough mixture, or a vaporizer, can be used.

If you run a high fever and are more than mildly ill, if the sputum becomes pus-laden indicating a possible bacterial infection on top of the original infection, or if there are other complicating factors, you should consult a physician. A suitable antibiotic may be needed.

Note: Although bronchitis is commonly a mild disease in a normally healthy person, it can be serious enough to warrant immediate attention in someone who is elderly, is debilitated for any reason, or has chronic lung or heart disease.

Bruises (Contusions)

In a bruise, or contusion, usually the result of a blow with a blunt object, there is no break in the skin but small blood vessels under the skin are ruptured and the internal bleeding is manifested in the typical black-and-blue mark.

WHAT TO DO: Minor bruises heal without special treatment. Applications of cold packs or ice in a towel, though, will help diminish the swelling, reduce pain caused by the swelling, and speed healing.

In healing, as blood is reabsorbed, the skin color gradually changes over a period of about two or three weeks from blue to green to yellow to normal.

If pain persists for more than a day, hot applications—hot water bottle, heating pad, or a warm-water-soaked towel—can help (but do not apply heat in the first 24 hours, as it may increase swelling).

If a bruise is very severe or if the blow was very forceful and the bruise is immediately over a bone, there is a possibility that the bone may have been fractured, and an x-ray probably will be needed.

Bursitis (See also ELBOW, TENNIS)

A bursa is a small sac or pouch located around a joint. It contains fluid and aids in making joint motion smooth and gliding. Bursae are found throughout the body, but the most important to you are those in the shoulder, elbow, knee, and hip.

In bursitis, a bursa becomes inflamed, sometimes as a result of gout. By far the most common cause, however, is excessive or improper use of the joint. Most often affected are the bursae deep in the shoulder, but almost any bursa in any joint in the body may become inflamed. Some of these inflammatory conditions have earned special names such as "housemaid's knee" and "tailor's bottom."

Bursitis produces great pain when any effort is made to move the joint. The joint area is tender and warm. When inflamed, the wall of a bursa secretes fluid; and if the bursa is superficial (near the surface of the body), swelling and redness often are apparent. Muscles in the area are tense and spastic, contracting involuntarily.

WHAT TO DO:

1. The first thing to do is to rest the joint on a pillow or in a sling.
2. To help relieve the pain, you can take aspirin (or, if you are sensitive to aspirin, an equivalent such as acetaminophen).
3. To help minimize the swelling, apply cold compresses or ice packs the first day. On the second day, moist, warm (not hot) applications help.
4. Once acute pain subsides, use gentle exercises for the joint in order to prevent adhesions, which can lead to chronic disability.

If the pain is severe, fails to yield in a few days, or if because of your job or for another reason it is important to try to speed relief right from the beginning, your family physician—or an orthopedic or other specialist to whom he may refer you—can help.

Sometimes, the physician may prescribe an antiinflammatory drug, phenylbutazone, to be taken by mouth for five days; it may provide gratifying relief.

Or, under local anesthesia, the physician may reach the inflamed bursa with a needle, withdraw some of the fluid, and instill a corticosteroid, or cortisone-like drug. Sometimes such treatment can produce almost immediate relief. Unfortunately, however, sometimes insertion of the needle may intensify the pain.

CHRONIC BURSITIS: This may develop when acute bursitis fails to clear completely or there are repeated attacks of acute bursitis. Movement of the joint then may become limited, and there may be flare-ups of pain similar to attacks of acute bursitis. Calcium deposits may collect in the bursa.

Chronic bursitis is treated in the same way as acute except that calcium deposits may have to be removed by surgery or by drawing them out through a large needle (aspiration). If adhesions also are present, physical therapy is needed.

Canker Sores (Aphthous Stomatitis)

These acute, painful ulcers of the mouth occur singly or in groups, and recurrent attacks are common. They last, in their acutely painful phase, 3 or 4 days, after which they heal in 7 to 10 days.

The cause is not certain. A wide variety of measures have been used with varying success. Rinsing the sores with a weak solution of sodium bicarbonate may lessen the pain. A commercial preparation containing sodium perborate is available from your druggist; and used as a mouth rinse as directed, it is sometimes effective in quickly eliminating small sores. A topical anesthetic such as 2 percent lidocaine (viscous), one tablespoonful, as an oral rinse every three hours or before meals may provide short-term relief and make it easier to eat.

If you suffer repeatedly from severe canker sores, your physician may decide to prescribe an oral suspension of an antibiotic. It is held in the mouth, in a dose of 250 milligrams, for two to five minutes to coat the sores, then is swallowed, and is usually used this way four times a day for four days. According to some trials, one antibiotic in particular, tetracycline, is more effective than any other measure if started soon after onset of the sores, often relieving symptoms during the first day and aborting new sores. It must be repeated for each attack.

Carbuncle (See BOILS AND CARBUNCLES)

Chafing (Intertrigo)

Chafing, an irritation of the skin also known as intertrigo, is the result of friction from clothing or the rubbing together of body surfaces such as thighs when they are damp from perspiration. Tight shoes, poorly fitting brassieres, and other items of clothing that bind may be responsible for chafing. Babies are particularly susceptible.

WHAT TO DO: You can usually clear up the irritation by keeping the areas dry. Applying a plain talcum powder often helps. By all means, if you can, substitute clothing that does not bind or rub. In the acute phase, you can place a dry sterile gauze pad over the area to prevent clothes from touching it. Remove the dressing and expose the chafed skin to the air when clothes are not being worn.

Chalazion (See EYELID CYST OR TUMOR)

Chest Injury (See also FRACTURES, DISLOCATIONS, STRAINS, AND SPRAINS)

Even without fracture of a rib or the breastbone, a heavy blow to the chest may lead to internal injuries. Ribs are flexible, particularly in young people, and although ribs may not be broken, the chest may be compressed enough to break blood vessels or damage the lungs or heart. This is a particular risk in automobile accidents in which the driver is thrown against the steering wheel.

If there is breathing difficulty, persistent chest pain, or marked restlessness after a heavy blow or series of blows to the chest, treat for shock (see p. 28) and get medical help to establish what internal damage has occurred and what must be done to repair it.

Chickenpox (See CHILDHOOD DISEASES, COMMUNICABLE)

Childbirth

Birth, of course, is a natural process. Although it involves labor for the mother, it goes forward without complications in the overwhelming majority of cases.

And if you ever must aid in a birth that occurs without benefit of physician or hospital, chances are great that you can do so successfully.

UNDERSTANDING THE PROCESS: On average, a woman having her first baby will feel mild labor twinges about 15 or 16 hours before delivery. With successive babies, that time may be halved.

There are three stages of labor.

Stage one, dilation, is usually the longest, although it can vary greatly in length. In this stage, the cervix, or mouth of the uterus, gradually dilates from a small opening to about four inches, in order to allow passage of the baby's head. Labor pains, or contractions, are caused by the tightening and relaxation of the muscles pulling the cervix open. The contractions increase in frequency, usually occurring at first at 10-minute intervals, then gradually progressing to every 4 minutes, 3 minutes, 2 minutes, to 1 minute or a little less. Each contrac-

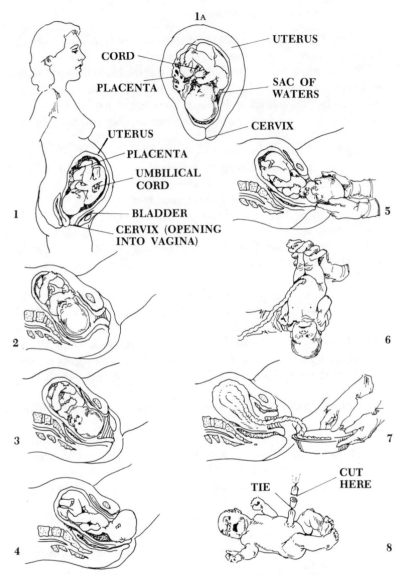

Fig. 12. Birth of a baby. 1 and 1A: Child in uterus near term. 2, 3, 4: The baby's head emerges. 5: The head turns to permit shoulders to emerge. 6: Raising the baby to permit mucus to drain from chest and throat. 7: Expulsion of the placenta (afterbirth). 8: Tying and cutting the cord.

tion usually lasts 20 to 60 seconds, and contraction strength gradually increases as the cervix opens.

The contractions are involuntary; the mother does not have to, and should not try to, bear down, but rather should relax as much as possible during the early first stage. And to help, you can provide reassurance and make her as comfortable as possible.

Stage two, expulsion or delivery, may take up to two hours for a first child, one-fourth that time or even less for a later one. Now, with the cervix completely dilated, the baby is ready to slide down into the vagina or birth canal.

At this point, because of the pressure of the baby's head on the rectum, the mother may feel as though she needs to have a bowel movement. But she must not go to the bathroom or she risks having the baby in the toilet. Explain the reason for the feeling and reassure her.

Delivery is close at hand when strong labor pains are coming 1 to 3 minutes apart and a bulge appears at the vaginal entrance. Now the mother should try to bear down with each contraction. She should be lying on her back with knees drawn up. (In some Asiatic countries, the mother gets on her hands and knees, allowing gravity to aid in the baby's passage.)

Although the bag of waters may break at any time during the first or second stage, it usually does so at the beginning of the second stage. Up to a quart of fluid and blood-stained mucus may either seep out or be expelled forcefully. This is expected; do not be alarmed by it.

We'll discuss the *third stage*, expulsion of the placenta, or afterbirth, shortly.

WHAT TO DO: If possible, wash your hands and see that the area around the mother is as clean as you can make it. Use clean sheets if available. Do not attempt to hurry or interfere with the birth.

In a normal delivery, the first sign of the baby usually will be the top of the head beginning to appear with each contraction. This is called "crowning," and once it occurs the baby will usually deliver within the next two or three contractions.

The head should not be allowed to pop out too quickly. By

placing your hand gently on the baby's head, you can help to assure slow emergence with each contraction. Don't attempt to hold the baby back, however.

As the baby's head emerges, it is usually with face downward, but then there is quick rotation to face the mother's thigh in order for the shoulder to be delivered. (Remember that the vaginal opening is oval, with the long diameter running in the longitudinal axis of the body.)

About one minute after the head is delivered, another contraction will cause delivery of the shoulders and rest of body. If, as happens only occasionally, there should be some difficulty with shoulder delivery, you may be able to help to some extent. Usually the top shoulder appears first, and a very gentle downward pressure on the baby's head toward the floor will help bring the shoulder out. Thereafter, a slight upward pressure on the baby's head may help bring out the other shoulder. Once the shoulders are out, the rest of the body follows quickly and easily.

Two things to note: During the delivery process, support the baby on your arms to prevent its falling. And after the head appears, check to see if the cord is wrapped around the neck; if it is, quickly loosen it or slip it over the baby's head to avoid risk of strangling.

Usually, the baby will start to breathe and cry within two or three minutes. Holding the infant securely by the ankles and back, raise his body enough to permit mucus to drain from chest and throat. Wipe his mouth with gauze or a clean cloth, and pull the tongue gently forward to open the airway.

To help get the baby breathing, do not slap but rather stroke the back vigorously or stroke upward from the bottom of the neck toward the chin. Tapping the soles of the feet can also be tried. It may be necessary also to clean out mucus from the mouth and nose.

If breathing still does not start—and it is rare for an infant not to breathe quickly on his own after an emergency delivery —cover the baby's mouth and nose with your mouth and puff gently and briefly, at a rate of about 20 a minute. Usually the baby will breathe after a few puffs.

Place the child between the mother's thighs and cover to

keep him warm. There is no need to cut the umbilical cord until the *placenta*, or *afterbirth*, is expelled.

The *third stage*, expulsion of the placenta, usually occurs within a few minutes after the baby is delivered. Contractions, which stopped after the birth, start up again to expel the placenta. It will appear very bloody, and this is normal. Do not try to hurry the expulsion process by pulling on the cord or placenta. You can gently massage the mother's abdomen to help the uterus to contract. Contraction diminishes bleeding.

If the mother bleeds after the placenta is expelled, use a sanitary napkin to help absorb the blood. Also to help the uterus to contract and stop the bleeding, massage it through the abdominal wall, gently kneading until it feels firm. As long as an hour of the kneading may be required, and it should be continued until medical help arrives or the hospital is reached. Wrap the placenta in a towel and retain it so it can be checked by a doctor to make certain all of it has been expelled.

Cutting the cord: There is no urgency about this. In no circumstances should the cord be cut until it has stopped pulsating, which usually happens about five minutes after delivery.

To sever the cord, first, using clean cloth strips or tape, tie a square knot reinforced with an extra tie around the cord about four inches from the baby's abdomen, and tie another reinforced knot about two inches farther away. Tie the knots securely so there is no danger of the baby hemorrhaging when the cord is cut.

Cut between the two knots, using a scissors, knife, or other sharp clean instrument which has been immersed in boiling water or soaked in alcohol. Cover the cord end on the baby with a sterile dressing.

Keep mother and baby warm. Notify the mother's obstetrician or other physician. And take mother and child to a hospital. If the baby gurgles or develops difficulty in breathing, there is likely to be some mucus collected in his nose and mouth. Wipe it out with a cloth or, if necessary, with your finger. Or suck it out with a straw or something similar.

IN CASE OF COMPLICATION: If, instead of the baby's head, you see an arm or leg emerging first, cover with a clean towel and get the mother to a physician or hospital as quickly as possible. The baby may be lying crosswise in the uterus or one leg may be trapped. The physician will need to use instruments for delivery or a cesarean section may be required.

In a *footling presentation*, both feet appear first during delivery. In a *breech presentation*, the buttocks appear first. In both presentations, delivery is usually slow and a hospital can be reached in time. Footling and breech births are not as seriously complicated as often thought. A major problem in both is the possibility that the child's head may press the cord during delivery and impair flow of oxygen.

If there is delay in getting to a hospital, have the mother assume a knee-chest position (on her hands and knees instead of on her back). This helps delivery by adding body weight to gravity.

Often the first sign that there will be a breech delivery is the baby's dark green feces coming out the vagina. Usually, the mother can bear down with the contractions and the baby will emerge up to its navel. When this point is reached, you can try to assist with further delivery or, if you have doubts, can support the baby and get the mother to a hospital.

Often, when the baby is small, the mother may be able to go on by herself to complete the delivery. But if it takes more than a couple of contractions for delivery from the baby's navel to armpit, assistance may be needed. It will be necessary to bring out the arms before the head. Slide two fingers up along the upper arm of the baby, and, grasping the arm, slide it down across the chest and out. Do the same for the other arm. Next insert a finger into the baby's mouth and gently bring the chin down toward its chest so the head will deliver. If the head fails to emerge, you must make it possible for air to get to the baby without delay. Insert your index and middle fingers into the vagina, separate the sides of the fingers around the baby's nose and push up to free the face from the wall of the vagina. Maintain this position until a physician can finish the delivery.

If the umbilical cord should be delivered before the baby's head, compression of the cord could deprive the baby of oxygen. To prevent the compression, have the mother assume the knee-chest position, which shifts the weight of the baby off the cord. Or, alternatively, elevate the mother's hips and feet 12 to 16 inches; this may allow the baby to fall back into the uterus, taking pressure off the cord. If the cord is still exposed, cover gently with sterile dressing and take the mother to a hospital as fast as possible.

Another possibility, of course, is multiple birth. Don't get flustered. Use the same procedures as in normal delivery for each birth. Multiple birth babies are usually small, making delivery easy. After each delivery, tie the umbilical cord tightly; no need to cut it until both infants are delivered. If the second delivery is breech, follow the procedure for breech delivery just noted.

MISCARRIAGE: Although this may occur at any time, it usually happens during the first three and a half months of pregnancy. There may be either partial or complete expulsion, with bleeding and discharge of blood clots and tissue.

A woman who is miscarrying may appear to be in shock. Commonly, she is pale, perspiring, has a fast pulse, experiences abdominal cramps, is weak, and may not be able to stand. Calm and reassure her. Keep her quiet. Position her with hips and feet elevated 12 to 16 inches. Use sanitary napkins to absorb discharge fluid. Retain the napkins for medical study. And transport to a hospital as quickly as possible.

Childhood Diseases, Communicable

Four contagious viral diseases of childhood—chickenpox, mumps, measles, and German measles—are still common although there are effective vaccines for all but chickenpox. Hopefully, there will be greater use of the vaccines as there has been with vaccines for diphtheria, whooping cough, and tetanus.

Chickenpox

Recognizing it: After an incubation period of 2 to 3 weeks, chickenpox may begin with slight fever, headache, malaise, and occasionally sore throat. At about the same time, some-times a day or two later, a rash appears—small red spots, usu-ally first on the back and chest, then in crops elsewhere. After several hours the spots enlarge, and each develops a blister in the center filled with clear fluid, which turns yellow after a day or two. A crust or scab then forms and peels off in from 5 to 20 days, during which time there is severe itching.

Communicability: The period of contagion extends from about 2 days before the rash appears until all the crops have crusted over.

WHAT TO DO: Most cases of chickenpox are mild. Rarely are there any complications requiring medical help.

The child should be kept isolated, if possible, during the period of communicability.

Wet compresses can be used to help control itching. Cala-mine lotion also may help. If the itching is severe, you can contact your physician, who may prescribe an antihistamine to be taken by mouth or applied locally.

Because of the possibility of bacterial infection of the blis-ters if a child does much scratching, it is important to bathe the child often and wash his or her hands three or more times a day with soap and water. Clip the fingernails, too.

Scrupulous soap and water cleansing may combat a mild infection even if it starts. If, however, one or more of the blisters become infected enough to cause return of fever, your physician may need to prescribe an antibiotic.

Mumps

Recognizing it: After a 14- to 24-day incubation period, mumps begins with chilly sensations, headache, appetite loss, low to moderate fever, and malaise, which may last 12 to 24 hours before gland swelling appears. In mild cases, these early symptoms may be absent.

Pain with chewing or swallowing—especially of acidic fluids such as orange or lemon juice—is the first indication of gland involvement.

With *parotitis*—inflammation of the parotid salivary glands (one on each side of the face, just below and in front of the ear)—the swelling that is characteristic of mumps develops. The temperature then often rises to 103° or 104°F. Swelling reaches its peak about the second day and extends beyond the glands to the area further in front of and below the ears. Occasionally, other salivary glands—under the jaw and tongue —may be involved. The glands are extremely tender during the 1 to 3 days that fever is present.

Communicability: Although its communicability is less than that of chickenpox and measles, mumps is still quite contagious. The infection is spread by droplets of saliva or direct contact with materials contaminated by infected saliva. The viruses appear to gain access through the mouth. Communicability extends from about 2 days before first symptoms to disappearance of swelling.

WHAT TO DO: If at all possible, isolate the patient until gland swelling subsides. Any other children and young adults in the home who have not been vaccinated or have not had mumps should be watched closely. About 20 percent of susceptible boys past puberty, if they get the disease, will also develop *orchitis*, a painful complication affecting the testes but rarely causing sterility. They may possibly get some protection from mumps immune globulin if it is injected within the first few days after exposure. Involvement of the ovaries in postpubertal girls may occur occasionally but is less recognized and much less painful.

There is no drug to combat the virus, so treatment is directed at relieving symptoms. Postpubertal patients are best off in bed until fever is gone. A soft diet avoids some of the pain of chewing. Aspirin or acetaminophen may be used for headache and general discomfort.

Treatment for complications is also symptomatic. With orchitis, bed rest is needed. The physician may provide support for the scrotum in cotton on an adhesive-tape bridge between the thighs to minimize tension. Ice pack applications often help to relieve pain. If necessary, codeine as well as aspirin may be prescribed for pain relief.

The outlook for complete recovery in uncomplicated mumps is excellent. Even with complications, a permanent aftermath is rare.

Measles

Recognizing it: After an incubation period of 9 to 14 days, measles often begins with a tired feeling, fever, nasal discharge, hacking cough, and reddening of the eyes. In 2 to 4 more days, the characteristic *Koplik's spots*—fine white spots inside the mouth, usually opposite the first and second upper molar teeth—appear. They resemble tiny grains of white sand.

The typical rash usually appears 3 to 5 days after symptoms begin, usually 1 or 2 days after appearance of Koplik's spots. The rash consists of flat, pink, blotchy spots that begin in front of and below the ears and on the side of the neck. Within 24 to 48 hours, the rash spreads to the trunk and arms and legs, at which point the spots begin to fade on the face.

At the peak of the disease, temperature may go above 104°F, mild itching may be present along with swelling about the eyes, red eye, and sensitivity to light. In 3 to 5 days, fever falls, the patient is more comfortable, and the rash fades rapidly.

Communicability: Measles is communicable from 2 to 4 days before the appearance of the rash until 2 to 5 days after onset.

WHAT TO DO: Treatment is symptomatic. During fever, the patient should remain in bed to help avoid complications. Itching can be relieved with calamine lotion applied several times a day.

Patients with measles are susceptible to pneumonia, middle ear and other bacterial infections. They should be protected as much as possible from exposure to anyone else with any kind of illness. An exacerbation of fever and development of pain or prostration may indicate a complicating bacterial infection for which your physician will prescribe a suitable antibiotic.

German Measles

Recognizing it: Also known as *3-day measles* and *rubella,* German measles may begin after a 2- to 3-week incubation period with malaise and tender swelling of lymph nodes about the neck.

After 1 to 5 days, the rash appears. It is similar to that of measles but less extensive, begins on face and neck and quickly spreads to trunk and arms and legs. There are flat or slightly raised red spots which may merge into large patches. The rash usually lasts about 3 days and on the second day may be accompanied by a flush. As the rash fades, a slight skin discoloration remains but disappears after about a day.

Communicability: German measles is communicable from shortly before beginning of symptoms until the rash disappears. It is spread by airborne droplets or by close contact.

Note that German measles is less contagious than measles and many people are not infected during childhood. As a result, 10 percent or more of young adult women are susceptible, and if they are infected during pregnancy there is risk to the fetus. Vaccination is protective and is especially important for girls.

WHAT TO DO: Uncomplicated German measles usually requires no treatment. It is rarely necessary to use even aspirin for fever. Middle ear infection, a rare complication, should be treated with a suitable prescribed antibiotic.

LESS COMMON DISEASES

Two other contagious childhood diseases are roseola and scarlet fever. The agent responsible for roseola is unknown, although there is a suspicion it may possibly be a virus. Scarlet fever is caused by streptococcal bacteria.

Roseola

Recognizing it: Mainly a disease of infants and young children, roseola is believed to have an incubation period probably of 4 to 7 days.

It begins with a fever of 103° to 104° for several days. Then, on about the fourth day, the temperature drops suddenly to normal and a pink-reddish rash appears on chest and abdomen and mildly on the face, arms, and legs. The rash may last 1 to 2 days.

Communicability: The period of communicability for roseola is unknown.

WHAT TO DO: There is no specific drug for the disease. Aspirin and tepid water or alcohol sponge baths can be used to bring the fever below 103°. When the temperature becomes normal and the rash appears, the child is usually so nearly well that no further treatment is needed.

Scarlet Fever

Also known as *scarlatina,* scarlet fever, once very common, is no longer so, probably because of antibiotic treatment for other strep infections of the throat, skin, ear, or other part of the body which usually precede scarlet fever.

Recognizing it: After an incubation period of 1 to 7 days, variable symptoms appear. They may include sore throat and swelling of neck lymph nodes. The tonsils may be covered by a patchy, pus-laden discharge. A bright red rash appears on the second day and may be localized or widespread; it is usually best seen on the abdomen. In mild cases, the temperature may rise to 101°F; in severe, to as high as 105°. Headache, chills, and nausea may occur. The rash fades within a week.

Communicability: Usually from 24 hours before beginning of symptoms until 2 to 3 weeks later.

WHAT TO DO: Your physician should be consulted because a suitable antibiotic will speed disappearance of symptoms and also help to prevent complications such as abscessed tonsils, middle ear infection, sinusitis, and mastoiditis. Aspirin may also be used for fever or sore throat.

Cold, Common

The common cold remains a nuisance, still without any established effective preventive or cure. There are, however, some things you can do that may reduce risk of getting a cold and some others to make a cold, once present, somewhat more tolerable.

Also, there are guidelines for distinguishing between a cold and flu, strep throat, or other problems that may mimic the cold to a greater or lesser degree.

It's an old question: If we can put a man on the moon, why can't we prevent or cure a cold? A cold is a virus-caused catarrhal respiratory tract infection which can affect any or all airways, including nose, throat, larynx, and often the windpipe and bronchial tubes. Any of multitudinous viruses can cause a cold. There are, for example, more than 95 types of just one family of viruses (rhinovirus), which may be involved. This is apparently the reason why colds can occur so often, why you develop no natural immunity, and why vaccination or immunization continues to be impractical.

SYMPTOMS: Onset of a cold is usually abrupt, after an incubation period of 18 to 48 hours. Often, first indications are a scratchy throat sensation, followed by sneezing, copious running of the nose, and some degree of malaise (that "blah" feeling). Typically, there is no fever although in babies and small children a temperature of 100° to 102°F is common. Cough and headache may be present. Later the nose becomes stuffed and the voice may become weak and husky.

The sinuses may be involved, causing some sinus pain. Purulent sinusitis, with a pus-containing nasal discharge, is a bacterial complication of a cold.

Colds often last from 4 to 10 days, with symptoms gradually subsiding after about the fourth day, sometimes a little earlier.

DISTINGUISHING BETWEEN A COLD AND OTHER INFECTIONS: Flu begins like a cold, with nasal stuffiness, headache, cough, but soon the malaise and fever (up to 104°) become quite severe, with strong muscle aches in the back and legs. Like a cold, the flu is caused by several different viruses (see INFLUENZA).

Most sore throats are viral, like colds. But *strep throat,* a bacterial infection, may begin with cold symptoms. It is soon accompanied by chills, very sore throat, high fever, swallowing difficulty, rapid and sometimes irregular pulse. Accurate diagnosis of a strep throat requires a throat culture test, although obvious redness of the throat warrants a presumptive medical diagnosis of strep throat and calls for prescribed antibiotics. Suitable antibiotic treatment can be curative.

Some childhood diseases may briefly appear to be colds. For example, measles, German measles, and chickenpox can simulate a cold until the telltale body rash appears. Whooping cough, after early cold symptoms, leads to a severe cough which rapidly gets worse. Meningitis begins with cold symptoms that soon progress to high fever and a characteristic stiff neck.

WHAT TO DO FOR A COLD:

1. First, do no harm. Antibiotics are of no value against the viruses of a cold and may make matters worse by producing side reactions, including digestive upsets.

2. Relieve symptoms as necessary. Aspirin or other antipain, antifever drug such as acetaminophen can be useful for relieving headache and fever. Two 5-grain tablets can be used if needed every four hours. Note that aspirin or another agent for pain and fever is not essential, does nothing to end a cold, and so need not be taken as a matter of course if you have no fever and are not especially bothered by headache.

3. Steam inhalations can help relieve chest tightness.

4. For a sore throat, a warm salt-water gargle every three or four hours can be soothing. Use one or two teaspoons of salt in a glass of water.

5. For a stuffed or running nose, long-acting "cold" pills are effective though not inexpensive and contain many ingredients, some of which may be of little or no value. Many contain an antihistamine, for example, which is of use only if the nose is running because of allergy. An antihistamine is likely to make you drowsy. For a stuffed nose, a simple nose drop preparation (one is Neo-Synephrine) is effective. Use it no more often than every 3 or 4 hours, and stop using it just as soon as you can do without it, since prolonged use may cause a rebound reaction and increased stuffiness. *Never use such drugs if you have a heart condition or high blood pressure.*

6. For a nose made tender by blowing, use any simple ointment containing petrolatum.

7. Bed rest can be important if the cold is heavy or if fever is present, especially for children. No adult without fever is likely to stay in bed, and need not, but getting as much rest as possible is helpful. So is an adequate intake of fluids, all kinds.

Do not try sweating out a cold by hot baths or heavy exercise, which may only weaken the body and make you more susceptible to complicating secondary infection.

It's a good idea to take temperature a few times a day. If temperature should go up, especially past 101°F, your doctor should be consulted because of the possibility of a bacterial complication, which can be treated with an antibiotic. Also check with a physician if you experience increasing chest pain, become short of breath when resting, cough up bloody mucus, wheeze, or if cough persists more than a week.

VITAMIN C: The debate about vitamin C's value in preventing or shortening colds still goes on. Some studies indicate value; others fail to find any.

According to Dr. Linus Pauling, the original proponent, a gram or more a day of vitamin C will block most but not all colds. If you feel tired or listless or are under some strain, he advises taking one or two grams more and continuing that amount every hour until you feel better. It is, he says, especially important to begin this high hourly intake at the very first sign of a cold—the first sneeze, shiver, or drop of nasal secretion. If you do, he has reported, usually your body can stop the cold, and even if it is not stopped, the high intake of vitamin C (totaling 10 to 30 grams a day) will ameliorate it so greatly you will have much less discomfort and be less likely to contract a secondary bacterial infection.

Pauling also advises that the best kind of vitamin C to use is the cheapest—pure crystalline powder vitamin C or 1-gram tablets. No need for more expensive rose-hip or acerola vitamin C.

PREVENTION: SOME NEW INSIGHTS: The usual advice for trying to minimize the risk of getting a cold has been to avoid crowds in winter and stay as far away as you can from coughers and sneezers. It may still be worthwhile to follow that advice if possible, but here are two newer insights into the problem of cold spread.

bacco—exacerbate your problem, you would, of course, be well advised to try limiting or eliminating them.

You might also try a high-fiber diet for, say, a month to see if it makes a considerable difference for you. Such a diet could include a bran or other cereal which is not highly refined, perhaps an increase in vegetable intake (vegetables are rich in fiber), and perhaps too some miller's bran.

Since irritable colon can imitate much more serious intestinal conditions, it is wise to have a thorough examination to rule out other disease. With that done and your mind at ease, relatively simple, drugless treatment may be sufficient.

Coma, Diabetic (See DIABETIC REACTIONS)

Conjunctivitis (See EYE, RED)

Constipation

Constipation is one of the most common human complaints —not always justified, often misunderstood and mistreated, only occasionally associated with a serious organic problem.

It is even variously defined. Many people believe that a daily bowel movement is normal and essential. It may be normal for some people but is not necessarily essential: some people go through life having no more than two, three, or four movements a week and have no problems—and don't consider that they do, nor do physicians. Some people believe that a stool must have a certain color or consistency; not so. Because of mistaken beliefs, the human colon is heavily abused with laxatives, suppositories, and enemas.

Constipation can arise from such organic causes as a debilitating infection or a thyroid or adrenal gland disorder—and there will then be other symptoms. When stools become thin

Not long ago, University of Wisconsin investigators were surprised by a study they carried out that indicated that the prevailing idea that the common cold spreads like wildfire from person to person may be as much of a myth as the old belief that wet feet and chill make for colds.

They found 24 couples, most of them students at the university, who volunteered to risk a cold in the interest of science. One person in each couple was infected by instilling nose drops containing a cold virus. As expected, the infected people came down with colds.

But only 38 percent transmitted their colds to their spouses. In the cases of transmission, the original cold was moderate or severe rather than mild in symptoms and the transmission took a lot of extended close contact: where the spouses became infected, the couples spent more than 17 hours a day together.

Another study, at the University of Virginia, indicates that colds are much more likely to be transmitted by fingers or hands—by direct skin-to-skin contact or even by touching surfaces contaminated by cold virus—than by sneeze or cough.

The study found that in only 2 of 25 people with naturally acquired colds was any virus expelled in a cough or sneeze. On the other hand, 40 percent of those with colds shed viruses onto their hands.

Moreover, viruses on hands could be transmitted to almost anything touched. The investigators were able to recover active viruses for up to three hours after they were deposited on wood, stainless steel and Formica surfaces and on such synthetic fabrics as Dacron and nylon. The viruses seemed to last less long on porous fabrics such as facial tissue and cotton cloth.

Drying had little effect on the viability of the viruses. Four of 11 people got colds after touching their nasal mucosa with fingers that had rubbed a dried drop of virus.

The investigators also observed, without being noticed, several hundred adults—doctors and medical students attending a lecture, another group of people in Sunday school. The object: to check on nose-picking and eye-rubbing. Per hour of observation, 1 of every 3 subjects picked his nose and 1 of every 2.7 rubbed his eyes. Incidentally, the observers noted that physicians and medical students picked their noses nine times more often than the Sunday school attendees, but both groups rubbed their eyes with equal frequency.

The study thus suggests that especially when a cold appears in a family, its spread might well be avoided by avoidance of eye-rubbing and nose-picking, and that hand-washing may be more important than covering up coughs and sneezes.

Cold Exposure (See FROSTBITE)

Cold Sores (See FEVER BLISTERS)

Colitis, Mucous (See COLON, IRRITABLE)

Colon, Irritable

A very common problem, irritable colon is also known by such names as *irritable bowel, spastic colon,* and *mucous colitis.* Colitis is a misnomer since it implies inflammation; there is no inflammation in the irritable bowel syndrome. Also, irritable colon is not to be confused with ulcerative colitis, which can be a serious condition.

The symptoms are extremely variable. If you have an irritable bowel problem, you may experience attacks of abdominal distention or bloating and pain, which may be sharp or deep and dull. You may even develop cramps which, when they occur on the right side, can be similar to those of appendicitis.

Often, victims suffer from constipation, sometimes from constipation alternating with diarrhea. Excess mucus may appear in stools.

Some victims complain of lack of appetite in the m nausea, heartburn, excessive belching—and, not monly, weakness, faintness, palpitation, and headache

There have been many theories about cause. One most popular is that emotional stress is a prime fact many victims are, in fact, tense and anxious, given tional lability, often to overwork, hurried and irregula and abuse of laxatives.

A new, more recent theory holds that the colon necessarily be irritable but rather may be irritated by diet, which tends to be soft and fiberless, with virt natural dietary fiber removed from breakfast cereals ar used for breads, cakes, and pastries.

To be sure, some blame has been placed on diet in and there are patients whose symptoms seem to be bated by very hot or very cold drinks, coffee, and alco

The newer theory holds that lack of dietary fiber is tant for many if not most people with irritable colon. A have been recent reports, in both England and the States, that many people respond well to a high-fiber need nothing more. In one study, for example, 88 per group of patients with irritable colon benefitted m within three weeks after being asked to include 8 to spoons of bran a day, sprinkled on cereals and used ing. *Bran* is the part of the cereal removed in con milling—except in a few cereals such as shredded wh in cereals that have the word "bran" in their name also be purchased as miller's bran in health food stor more and more supermarkets stocking it.

WHAT TO DO: For one thing, you should realize th ble colon is extremely common, not caused by dise while distinctly uncomfortable, not a serious conditio

Conventional treatment has included use of mild se tranquilizers, and drugs such as belladonna and which provide symptomatic relief although often at pense of very dry mouth and vision disturbances. well be better off without medications and their side your symptoms are not very severe.

If you find that hot or cold drinks, coffee, alcohol—

Not long ago, University of Wisconsin investigators were surprised by a study they carried out that indicated that the prevailing idea that the common cold spreads like wildfire from person to person may be as much of a myth as the old belief that wet feet and chill make for colds.

They found 24 couples, most of them students at the university, who volunteered to risk a cold in the interest of science. One person in each couple was infected by instilling nose drops containing a cold virus. As expected, the infected people came down with colds.

But only 38 percent transmitted their colds to their spouses. In the cases of transmission, the original cold was moderate or severe rather than mild in symptoms and the transmission took a lot of extended close contact: where the spouses became infected, the couples spent more than 17 hours a day together.

Another study, at the University of Virginia, indicates that colds are much more likely to be transmitted by fingers or hands—by direct skin-to-skin contact or even by touching surfaces contaminated by cold virus—than by sneeze or cough.

The study found that in only 2 of 25 people with naturally acquired colds was any virus expelled in a cough or sneeze. On the other hand, 40 percent of those with colds shed viruses onto their hands.

Moreover, viruses on hands could be transmitted to almost anything touched. The investigators were able to recover active viruses for up to three hours after they were deposited on wood, stainless steel and Formica surfaces and on such synthetic fabrics as Dacron and nylon. The viruses seemed to last less long on porous fabrics such as facial tissue and cotton cloth.

Drying had little effect on the viability of the viruses. Four of 11 people got colds after touching their nasal mucosa with fingers that had rubbed a dried drop of virus.

The investigators also observed, without being noticed, several hundred adults—doctors and medical students attending a lecture, another group of people in Sunday school. The object: to check on nose-picking and eye-rubbing. Per hour of observation, 1 of every 3 subjects picked his nose and 1 of every 2.7 rubbed his eyes. Incidentally, the observers noted that physicians and medical students picked their noses nine times more often than the Sunday school attendees, but both groups rubbed their eyes with equal frequency.

The study thus suggests that especially when a cold appears in a family, its spread might well be avoided by avoidance of eye-rubbing and nose-picking, and that hand-washing may be more important than covering up coughs and sneezes.

Cold Exposure (See FROSTBITE)

Cold Sores (See FEVER BLISTERS)

Colitis, Mucous (See COLON, IRRITABLE)

Colon, Irritable

A very common problem, irritable colon is also known by such names as *irritable bowel, spastic colon,* and *mucous colitis.* Colitis is a misnomer since it implies inflammation; there is no inflammation in the irritable bowel syndrome. Also, irritable colon is not to be confused with ulcerative colitis, which can be a serious condition.

The symptoms are extremely variable. If you have an irritable bowel problem, you may experience attacks of abdominal distention or bloating and pain, which may be sharp or deep and dull. You may even develop cramps which, when they occur on the right side, can be similar to those of appendicitis.

Often, victims suffer from constipation, sometimes from constipation alternating with diarrhea. Excess mucus may appear in stools.

Some victims complain of lack of appetite in the morning, nausea, heartburn, excessive belching—and, not uncommonly, weakness, faintness, palpitation, and headaches.

There have been many theories about cause. One of the most popular is that emotional stress is a prime factor. And many victims are, in fact, tense and anxious, given to emotional lability, often to overwork, hurried and irregular meals, and abuse of laxatives.

A new, more recent theory holds that the colon may not necessarily be irritable but rather may be irritated by modern diet, which tends to be soft and fiberless, with virtually all natural dietary fiber removed from breakfast cereals and flours used for breads, cakes, and pastries.

To be sure, some blame has been placed on diet in the past, and there are patients whose symptoms seem to be exacerbated by very hot or very cold drinks, coffee, and alcohol.

The newer theory holds that lack of dietary fiber is the irritant for many if not most people with irritable colon. And there have been recent reports, in both England and the United States, that many people respond well to a high-fiber diet and need nothing more. In one study, for example, 88 percent of a group of patients with irritable colon benefitted markedly within three weeks after being asked to include 8 to 10 teaspoons of bran a day, sprinkled on cereals and used in cooking. *Bran* is the part of the cereal removed in commercial milling—except in a few cereals such as shredded wheat and in cereals that have the word "bran" in their names. It can also be purchased as miller's bran in health food stores, with more and more supermarkets stocking it.

WHAT TO DO: For one thing, you should realize that irritable colon is extremely common, not caused by disease, and, while distinctly uncomfortable, not a serious condition.

Conventional treatment has included use of mild sedatives, tranquilizers, and drugs such as belladonna and atropine, which provide symptomatic relief although often at the expense of very dry mouth and vision disturbances. You may well be better off without medications and their side effects if your symptoms are not very severe.

If you find that hot or cold drinks, coffee, alcohol—and to-bacco—exacerbate your problem, you would, of course, be well advised to try limiting or eliminating them.

You might also try a high-fiber diet for, say, a month to see if it makes a considerable difference for you. Such a diet could include a bran or other cereal which is not highly refined, perhaps an increase in vegetable intake (vegetables are rich in fiber), and perhaps too some miller's bran.

Since irritable colon can imitate much more serious intestinal conditions, it is wise to have a thorough examination to rule out other disease. With that done and your mind at ease, relatively simple, drugless treatment may be sufficient.

Coma, Diabetic (See DIABETIC REACTIONS)

Conjunctivitis (See EYE, RED)

Constipation

Constipation is one of the most common human complaints —not always justified, often misunderstood and mistreated, only occasionally associated with a serious organic problem.

It is even variously defined. Many people believe that a daily bowel movement is normal and essential. It may be normal for some people but is not necessarily essential: some people go through life having no more than two, three, or four movements a week and have no problems—and don't consider that they do, nor do physicians. Some people believe that a stool must have a certain color or consistency; not so. Because of mistaken beliefs, the human colon is heavily abused with laxatives, suppositories, and enemas.

Constipation can arise from such organic causes as a debilitating infection or a thyroid or adrenal gland disorder—and there will then be other symptoms. When stools become thin and pencil-like and the change is accompanied by weight loss, a bowel tumor may be present. In the late stages of pregnancy, pressure of the fetus on the large bowel may produce constipation. When constipation is accompanied by swelling of the abdomen and abdominal pain, bowel obstruction is possible.

Certainly, if you have any reason to suspect an organic cause, you should see a physician for a rectal examination and a visual examination of the lower colon through a tubelike instrument, the *sigmoidoscope*. Newer sigmoidoscopes—made of flexible fiberoptic bundles—cause no discomfort. Sometimes, x-ray study may be needed.

But by far the vast majority of cases of constipation—*simple* constipation as it is called medically—stem from two causes.

One is failure to respond to the urge to evacuate the bowel. Sometimes, especially when traveling, it may be impossible to respond promptly. If this persists, constipation may follow. A good way to relieve it, in addition to eating properly and drinking plenty of fluids, is to engage in regular daily physical activity such as walking. And if you have been cooped up in a car, boat, plane, or train all or much of the day, a good long walk when you reach your destination will help.

The other problem is diet. Our highly refined diet today is a common reason for constipation. Fiber, a natural constituent, is processed out of many of our cereals and flours and the foods made from them. Fiber is vitally important, not as a nutrient (it has little nutritional value and very little is absorbed), but because it absorbs moisture in the gastrointestinal tract and in doing so gives bulk to the stool. When adequate fiber is eaten, stools are no longer hard and pebbly but soft and well-formed. It is easier for the muscles of the colon to move them along and easier for you to pass them out. With adequate fiber, it is highly likely that you can establish pleasant, easy regularity.

WHAT TO DO: Eating more fruits and vegetables—raw when that's palatable, lightly cooked otherwise—can increase fiber intake, but vegetables and fruits do contain varying amounts. There is, naturally, no fiber in meat, fish, fats, milk, sugar, or alcoholic drinks.

Seeds such as whole sesame and sunflower, along with

seed-filled berries such as raspberries, blackberries, and loganberries, are rich in dietary fiber.

Some, but far from all, breakfast cereals are rich in fiber. The rich: oatmeal (the old-fashioned, slow-cooking kind, not the "instant"); whole-grain wheat cereals designed to be cooked; shredded wheat; cereals labeled as "all bran" or made up of substantial amounts of bran.

You can substitute bread made from whole wheat or whole rye flour for white bread. Note that many brown breads are not whole meal, so don't depend on color alone but check the labeling (and if necessary the manufacturer) to find out whether bread is in fact made from whole wheat or whole rye flour.

You can if you like (it is not essential if you follow the foregoing suggestions) add unprocessed bran to your diet. This is the fiber-rich bran removed during the heavy milling of refined flour. It can be added, a teaspoonful or two at a time, to cereals, soups, sauces, puddings, fruit juice, and to flour used in baking.

By all means, avoid chronic use of laxatives. They do not get at the cause of constipation. They may give you a "lazy" colon. Some may interfere with food absorption or cause skin rashes, or even contribute to hemorrhoids.

If you must have immediate relief from acute constipation, an enema may help. Or you can use a laxative such as Metamucil or mineral oil. Milk of magnesia is a satisfactory laxative but should not be used if you have pain in the abdomen, since it could cause perforation of an acute appendix or rupture of a blocked bowel if either should be present.

Contusions (See BRUISES)

Convulsion

A convulsion is an episode of involuntary jerking movements frequently with unconsciousness which may be momentary or may last several minutes.

Convulsions have many possible causes. They often occur in young children in association with high fever. They occur in some forms of epilepsy. Other causes include stroke, central nervous system infections (such as meningitis, encephalitis, brain abscess, rabies, and tetanus), metabolic disturbances such as hypoglycemia (low blood sugar), carbon monoxide poisoning, skull fracture, brain tumor, drug reaction, and withdrawal from alcohol, sleeping pills, or tranquilizers.

WHAT TO DO: Whatever the cause, the primary aim of emergency management is to prevent injury. If you can, insert a firm but relatively soft object, such as a folded handkerchief or a cloth wrapped around a toothbrush handle, between the teeth to protect the tongue. Loosen clothing around the neck. If you can manage it, place a pillow under the head.

While protecting the patient, seek medical help or take the victim to a hospital emergency room.

Convulsions in themselves rarely are fatal. The major risk associated with them is injury to mouth or head.

Croup

Croup, which can occur at any age but is far more common in children, especially those 6 months to 3 years of age, is very likely to cause anxiety for both child and parents.

Also known as *acute laryngotracheobronchitis*, which means inflammation of the larynx (voice box), trachea (windpipe), and bronchi (air passages from windpipe to lungs), it is an acute viral infection.

Typically, a child has a mild upper respiratory infection and mild temperature elevation followed by hoarseness and perhaps a "barking" cough. Then, usually late at night, the child wakes up because of trouble in breathing. There are harsh sounds upon inhaling.

Croup is most common in winter and spring.

WHAT TO DO: Because a child with croup is likely to be terrified at his breathing difficulty, it is essential for you to be calm yourself and to do everying possible to soothe and calm the child.

For immediate, emergency relief, take the child into the bathroom, close the door, and turn on hot water from all faucets to build up humidity quickly. Sit with the child, talk to him, tell him a story, until breathing improves.

If there is no improvement or if the child begins to develop a bluish color, indicating lack of adequate oxygen, call your physician or take the child immediately to a hospital emergency room.

In most cases, the child will be very much relieved by the steam treatment and able to go back to sleep afterward. Let him do so and get a vaporizer working in his room.

Undoubtedly, you will feel better—and often it is a good idea—if you stay in the child's room overnight and even for another two or three nights just in case of the possibility of another attack.

Make sure the child gets adequate fluids.

Very commonly, croup gets better with these simple measures.

In a very severe case of croup, hospital treatment can be effective. In the hospital, oxygen may be administered, as needed, by mask or tent, and nebulized mist may be used. Mist therapy helps to reduce the thickness of respiratory secretions and make them easier to eliminate through coughing. The viruses that most often cause croup usually do not predispose to a superimposed bacterial infection, but if that should occur, antibiotics can be used.

Cuts (Lacerations)

Most of the time, cuts affect just the skin and underskin fatty tissue and heal well without need for medical help.

WHAT TO DO: For such minor cuts, apply soap and water vigorously, and make certain no debris is left. You can then usually apply Band-Aids or strips of sterile paper tape so that the wound edges come together neatly and are held that way. Do not pull the edges together if the cut occurred more than three or four hours before.

When may medical help be needed?

If there are any indications of infection—pus, fever, marked redness and swelling (which, if they are going to appear, usually take at least 24 hours to do so)—a physician should be consulted.

If there are any indications of nerve or major blood vessel damage—numbness, tingling, weakness (in a cut arm or leg), or vigorous blood flow—medical help is needed.

A physician should be seen if, for any reason, the edges of a fresh cut—perhaps because they are jagged—cannot be brought together neatly.

Unless very minor, any facial laceration should be repaired by a physician, perhaps even by a surgeon, so as to minimize possibility of a disfiguring scar.

Any deep laceration of the hand should be looked at by a physician because of the possibility that nerves for sense of touch or tendons controlling finger movements may have been cut and need very precise repair.

A SPECIAL WORD ABOUT SUTURING: There seems to be a common impression that suturing, or stitching, is the optimal

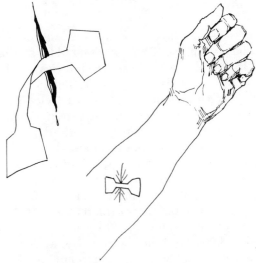

Fig. 13. Bringing edges of a cut together with tape.

way to repair a cut. That is not necessarily so. The only reason for suturing is to bring cut edges into contact so as to minimize scarring and promote healing or to control bleeding.

If a cut is not deep, if edges are not jagged and are close to each other, if no tendons, nerves or major blood vessels under the skin are involved, you can easily and effectively carry out the repair yourself by bringing the edges into contact and holding them there with tape or a few Band-Aids placed carefully across instead of lengthwise along the cut.

But, by all means, in other situations, or if you have doubts about how effectively you are repairing even a minor cut, see a physician.

See also scalp laceration under HEAD INJURIES.

Cystitis (See URINARY TRACT INFECTIONS)

Dehydration

Dehydration—in which excessive amounts of water are lost from the body—can result from prolonged fever, diarrhea, and vomiting. It may also occur in severe injuries involving loss of blood or body fluids. Heavy perspiration in hot weather or during a tennis game or other vigorous activity can be responsible. You may not see or feel the perspiration, particularly in hot, dry desert climate, but this unsensed perspiration can cause as much fluid loss as, or even more than, ordinary sweating. Overuse of diuretic drugs ("water pills"), which increase the volume of urine, also may lead to dehydration.

Water actually makes up more than half of body weight. Normally about two and a half quarts are lost daily through urination, in the stool, in exhaled breath, and by evaporation from the skin. Of course, the water carries away minerals such as salt and potassium. The loss is normally made up through liquids and minerals in foods.

Dehydration begins when losses exceed intake. Depending upon the degree of deficit, there may be one or more such symptoms as flushing, dry skin and mucous membranes, cracked lips, decreased urination, mental confusion, low blood pressure, muscle cramps, and even loss of consciousness.

WHAT TO DO: The first thing is to prevent a deficit. Fluids must be replenished. When exposed to any situation that can lead to dehydration, drink plenty of water, juice, broth, or other fluid. Since excessive loss of fluids may also mean loss of minerals, you may need to take at least some fluid with salt in it (half a teaspoonful to half a glass of water). Alcohol must be avoided since it has a dehydrating effect.

If nausea is present, an effort still must be made to get fluid down. Try very small sips—say, a teaspoonful—every five minutes or so. Sucking ice chips is also effective. For unknown reasons, cold colas and carbonated drinks can diminish nausea for many people and could be worth trying.

In severe dehydration, medical help is essential. Treatment may require replacement not only of fluid but also of specific vital minerals. Saline solutions, blood plasma, or whole blood may have to be injected.

Whether mild, moderate, or severe, dehydration must be treated for itself. But it is also essential to determine the cause and treat that if it is something other than a fleeting upset.

Note: Infants are particularly susceptible to easy dehydration. They have much less of a body reserve of fluid and can develop shock or lose consciousness rapidly. In severe cases accompanied by vomiting, a physician will have to replace the fluid and minerals by injection. Such injection has often saved the lives of desperately sick infants.

Delirium

A disordered mental state with excitement and illusions, delirium can be brought on by almost any acute illness accompanied by very high fever.

Other possible causes include physical and mental shock, exhaustion, head injury, liver or kidney failure, very low thyroid function, insufficient or excess blood sugar. Delirium also may occur in association with excessive intake of alcohol or sedatives, anesthesia, and following drug withdrawal (especially of alcohol and barbiturates).

Most cases of delirium begin fairly suddenly. There is clouding of consciousness along with confusion, disordered speech, difficulty in comprehension, sometimes lack of appreciation of time, place, and (in severe cases) person. There may be overwhelming fear; less commonly, elation or depression; occasionally, excitability, irritability, and violent behavior.

Delirium can be relatively brief (a matter of hours) or may last for weeks, often with fluctuations in which the patient appears better at times, worse at others. Commonly, the patient is worse during evenings and at night.

WHAT TO DO: Delirium requires medical attention as soon as possible. The outlook for recovery is good if the underlying condition can be reversed, as it often can be.

While waiting for medical help, approach the patient in a calm, reassuring manner. If possible, keep him in a quiet, nonstimulating environment. Keep the light dim but do not make the room totally dark. Watch closely to protect him from any self-injury. If necessary, restrain him by encircling his chest with a folded sheet; tie it under the bed. Should he endanger himself by flailing his arms, it may be necessary to tie each wrist, at his side, to the bed. Use sheets, not string or rope, which can cut off circulation or cut into the skin. Restraints should not be too tight; they should allow some movement. Be certain restraints are actually necessary; sometimes they can serve as an added exciting factor.

If you are far from medical help and there will be extended delay in obtaining it, try to see that the patient eats and drinks adequately. If possible, see to it that elimination from bowel and bladder is adequate.

If high fever is present, work on that. In addition to giving two aspirin tablets every three to four hours, sponge off the patient with lukewarm water or alcohol.

Only if there is likely to be extended delay in medical help and the patient is so disturbed as to make management difficult—and, of course, if you have any available—you can try giving a drug such as Valium or Thorazine. If you do have it, it will usually be in oral form and may help, although severely disturbed patients often require intramuscular injection of such agents.

Diabetic Reactions (Insulin Shock, Diabetic Acidosis/Coma)

Loss of effective control of diabetes, even a temporary loss, can lead to emergency reactions. In one reaction, the trouble lies with insulin in excess. In the other, insulin is inadequate.

Insulin Shock

This is a *hypoglycemic* (or low blood sugar) reaction. It can result from an overdose of insulin. But it can also commonly stem from lowered blood sugar caused by a departure from your usual routine. You may, for example, fail to eat a meal at the usual time, or engage in an unusual amount of exercise or physical activity, or have an emotional upset, or suffer from a change in body chemistry such as may be caused by infection.

SYMPTOMS: Insulin shock develops suddenly. Symptoms include weakness, moist and pale skin, with cold sweating and tremors. Manifestations may differ in some cases and can include nausea, dizziness, headache, and drowsiness. The pulse is quickened. There may be muscular spasms and emotional reactions such as excessive laughing or crying. Convulsions may occur and, ultimately, unconsciousness.

WHAT TO DO: A diabetic patient should be familiar with insulin shock symptoms long before they occur and at the very first indication of an attack should take some form of sugar. The sugar can be in lump form, or it can be taken by the spoonful, or it can be added to a glass of orange juice.

If you must help a diabetic in insulin shock, give sugar or a food rich in sugar such as candy. But if the patient is unconscious, do not force food or liquid; you may cause choking. Call a physician or emergency squad or take the person to a hospital emergency room.

Diabetic Acidosis/Coma

This reaction occurs when too much food or too little insulin is taken, or there is less than usual physical activity, so that sugar is not burned at the usual rate, builds up in the blood, and appears in the urine.

SYMPTOMS: Great thirst, dry skin and tongue, and flushing develop with acidosis. The pulse is weak and rapid. Fever may be present. Vomiting is common, and often there is abdominal pain. The breath may have the odor of acetone, a principal ingredient of fingernail polish remover.

Unlike insulin shock which develops suddenly, diabetic acidosis has a gradual onset over a period of days. If disregarded, it can lead to coma and sometimes even death.

A danger with coma is that it may be mistaken for drunkenness, and medical treatment for the coma may be neglected until too late.

If you are confronted with an unconscious person who is breathing (and therefore has not become unconscious due to choking), and if the cause of unconsciousness is unknown, smell the breath and suspect diabetic acidosis if you detect acetone. This may still be a difficult decision if the diabetic person has been drinking alcohol. Look for an identification tag that diabetics often carry to indicate their condition.

WHAT TO DO: Diabetic acidosis requires treatment with insulin and also with intravenous fluids. Immediate medical help is urgent.

For prevention, diabetics should, of course, take the proper dosage of insulin regularly. Also, they must avoid eating sprees and must watch for conditions that can require extra amounts of insulin, such as colds, other infections, dental extractions.

Differences Between Insulin Shock and Diabetic Acidosis

	Insulin shock	*Diabetic adidosis*
Cause	Too much insulin	Too little insulin
Onset	Sudden	Gradual
Food intake history	May be insufficient	Normal or excessive
Skin	Moist, pale	Dry, flushed
Mouth	Drooling	Dry
Thirst	Absent	Great
Hunger	Sometimes	Absent
Vomiting	Rare	Common
Abdominal pain	Absent	Frequent
Breathing	Normal or shallow	Exaggerated, deep, noisy
Pulse	Full, bounding	Weak, rapid
Treatment	Sugar to eat	Insulin injection

Diarrhea

Diarrhea—the repeated passage of unformed, watery stools —is only a symptom. It is common with "intestinal flu" or other viral disease of the intestinal tract. It can also be brought on by excessive alcohol intake, overindulgence in food, or emotional upset.

WHAT TO DO: Usually, diarrhea doesn't last long and can be treated readily at home. Because diarrhea can dehydrate, increase your intake of water and other fluids. Applesauce may help. So, too, a tablespoon of Kaopectate after each movement.

If these measures are not enough, an antidiarrheal agent containing paregoric is often effective. Paregoric (camphorated tincture of opium) has a soothing action on the bowel and allays griping pains. Some preparations contain, in addition to paregoric, kaolin to adsorb irritants and form a protective coating on the bowel lining, and pectin to consolidate the stool. The usual dosage of one such preparation, Parepectolin, is one or two tablespoons after each loose movement for no more than four doses in 12 hours. For children, one or two teaspoons after each loose movement for no more than four doses in twelve hours is usually recommended.

If diarrhea lasts more than a day or two, check with a physician. It may possibly indicate an ulcer, colitis, or other digestive tract disease.

Even early in a sudden bout of diarrhea, it can be important to check with a physician if you suspect bleeding from the bowel or experience not just the gaslike, cramping, on/off pains common with diarrhea but severe, steady or prolonged pain.

Another point to remember: Some drugs, although otherwise valuable, can cause diarrhea in some cases. If you have recently begun to use a new drug, including one prescribed by a physician, check with the physician for the possibility that it may be the reason for the diarrheal episode.

TRAVELER'S DIARRHEA: What causes *turista*, or traveler's diarrhea, has long been in doubt. But some recent studies indicate that certain organisms known as toxigenic *E. coli* are involved. These studies, which also looked into various medications that might possibly help, found that an old patent medicine, Pepto-Bismol, is often effective. Which of its ingredients combats turista is not clear, but an ounce every half hour for 4 hours has been reported to bring significant reduction in diarrhea, nausea, and cramps within 24 hours.

An even more recent study by the same investigators—of the University of Texas Medical School, Houston—has turned up evidence that Pepto-Bismol also can be effective in preventing turista. A study was carried out with 128 American students slated to attend classes in Guadalajara, Mexico. Diarrhea developed in only 14 of 62 who took four tablespoons of the preparation four times a day for 21 days beginning immediately upon arriving in Guadalajara. In contrast, it occurred in 40 of 66 students who, for comparison purposes, received a lookalike but inert preparation.

There has also been another promising development for protection against turista among those who visit developing countries. Although various antibacterial agents have been tried with only modest effects, recently doxycycline, an antibiotic, has been found useful. It's somewhat unusual as an antibiotic, too, in having a long-lasting effect, so that only a single 100-milligram daily dose is needed. In a study among Peace Corps volunteers in Kenya, doxycycline, when taken in advance, afforded protection in better than 90 percent of cases, and the protection seemed to last for at least a week after use was stopped. If you are going on a trip where turista may be a hazard, your physician may prescribe the antibiotic for you to take along.

Note: It is not very likely to happen, but if you should experience very severe diarrhea and medical help is not available, you may need to combat dehydration, manifested by extreme thirst and mouth and tongue dryness. If unchecked, it can be dangerous. To overcome the loss of both fluids and minerals, you can prepare a solution with one teaspoonful of table salt, one teaspoonful of baking soda, and four teaspoonsful of table sugar to a quart of water, adding flavoring if you like. This will help to restore both minerals and fluid. But get medical help as soon as possible.

Dislocations (See FRACTURES, DISLOCATIONS, SPRAINS, AND STRAINS)

Diverticular Disease

The word *diverticulum* means a pocket. In *diverticulosis*, the colon (large bowel) contains dozens, even scores of blind pouches or pockets formed as the colon lining pushes into and eventually through the bowel wall.

Diverticulosis itself produces no symptoms. It is present in more than one third of Americans over the age of 40.

But if fecal matter should become trapped in the pouches, inflammation and infection may develop, producing diverticulitis, a painful affliction.

Diverticulitis is sometimes referred to as "left-sided appendicitis" because of the similarity of its pain to that of the right-sided lower abdominal pain of appendicitis.

Diverticulitis attacks are severe, with the pain lasting minutes, hours or days, appearing at any time without relation to eating or activities. Other symptoms can include abdominal distention, nausea, occasionally vomiting, sometimes chills, fever, and malaise, or just a generally bad feeling.

WHAT TO DO: Bed rest and a liquid diet help during acute diverticulitis. Your physician may also prescribe an antibiotic to combat the infection. Usually, the infection and inflammation subside.

In a severe case, hospitalization and use of intravenous feeding may be tried in order to put the bowel at rest.

It is possible for a complication such as peritonitis (see p. 268) to develop, and this must be watched for and treated as an emergency if it should occur.

With repeated severe attacks or the development of complications, surgery may be needed. This consists of removing the portion of the large intestine that contains the pouches and joining the cut ends of intestine together to enable normal bowel function to be resumed.

This note of hope comes from recent studies: It appears that people who live on a high-fiber diet—vegetables, fruits, whole-grain breads and cereals—rarely get diverticular disease. A low-fiber diet produces small-volume stools, and to move such stools along, the colon must clamp down harder; the excessive clamping down leads to high pressures within the bowel that may account for the pushing out of the pouches. According to some recent medical reports, use of a high-fiber diet, once an acute attack of diverticulitis is over, may be of value in avoiding need for surgery.

Dizziness

Almost everyone has experienced the sensation of dizziness as a result of whirling around too fast or too long or perhaps while looking down from a great height. This sensation is markedly different from severe attacks of dizziness which physicians call *vertigo*.

It's important to distinguish the two if relief is to be obtained.

The first kind of dizziness is commonly described as a faint feeling, light-headedness, giddiness, or a kind of head-swimming sensation.

On the other hand, with true vertigo, you feel that you are being whirled about or that everything around you is whirling. In addition, you may be pale and sweaty, feel nauseated and may vomit, and may try to stay in one place because movement makes the symptoms worse. Vertigo also may sometimes be accompanied by ringing in the ears (*tinnitus*) or uncontrollable movements of the eyes (*nystagmus*).

It is not unusual for dizziness to occur with high fever or under other circumstances: when you have not eaten for a long time, or have smoked excessively, had too much to drink, or even when you get up very suddenly from a sitting or lying position so there is a momentary lapse in adequate blood supply to the brain.

Vertigo results from a disturbance somewhere in the balance or equilibratory apparatus, which consists of the labyrinth of the inner ear, areas of the brain, and the eyes.

These structures may be affected by any of a variety of disorders. Infections in or around the inner ear may lead to severe vertigo, as may bleeding into the labyrinth. Medicines such as quinine, salicylates (aspirin and aspirinlike compounds), and the antibiotic streptomycin, as well as opiates and alcohol, may sometimes set off vertigo by a toxic effect on the labyrinth. Motion sickness is a frequent cause. Brain or ear tumors, middle ear infection, and skull fracture can produce vertigo.

Meniere's disease, which involves faulty functioning of the labyrinth of the ear, is marked by attacks of true vertigo. In addition, there may be ringing in the ears and hearing impairment. Attacks last from a few minutes to several hours.

WHAT TO DO: For an occasional attack of dizziness that is not true vertigo, you can try drinking a glass of orange juice. Also, make it a practice to take it easy when getting up from a seated or lying-down position. One of the nonprescription antihistamine drugs sold for motion sickness may be helpful.

If dizziness is a recurring problem, it would be wise to have a physician check your blood pressure and examine your ear canals. He may also suggest other studies.

For true vertigo, you may get some relief from an attack with bed rest and an antihistamine. But don't leave it at that. Medical help is needed to determine and eliminate the cause —and even as the cause is sought and treated, the physician may prescribe more potent antihistamine or other medication to provide more effective relief for symptoms.

Dropsy (See EDEMA)

Drowning

Try to clear the airway as quickly as possible by turning the victim on his abdomen or lowering his head.

Recently, it has been shown that the Heimlich maneuver (p. 44) can evacuate water from the lungs, and therefore is an important first step in rescuing a drowning victim.

Follow immediately with mouth-to-mouth respiration (p. 49). If the heart has stopped beating, give complete cardio-pulmonary resuscitation (CPR) (p. 52).

If you find that mouth-to-mouth respiration is difficult or impossible, it could be because of debris or other obstruction. Surely, perform the Heimlich maneuver for choking, then proceed to respiration and, if necessary, complete CPR.

Persist with your efforts until help arrives. Many victims, seemingly beyond help, have been saved by extended efforts. Unlike choking victims, who can die within four minutes, drowning victims who have been submerged for half an hour have survived. This is particularly true if the water in which the drowning occurred is very cold, which diminishes the rate of metabolism, thus slowing up the use of oxygen still present in the body.

Dysentery, Amebic (See WORM-INDUCED DISEASES)

Dyspepsia (See INDIGESTION)

Earache

If you have an earache, pulling on the earlobe may help indicate whether there is infection in the outer ear canal or in the middle ear. If pain is intensified by pulling, the likelihood is that the problem lies in the outer ear canal.

Outer ear canal infection can occur at any time of year but is most common in summer during the swimming season and is often called *swimmer's ear*. Some people, particularly the allergic, are especially prone to such infections. Injury from trying to clean the ear canal with cotton-tipped sticks and the like can predispose to infection. Actually, the ear has its own cleansing mechanism, and your cleaning attempts may interfere with that mechanism, promoting accumulation of wax and debris behind which water can be trapped, setting the stage for infection.

An outer ear canal infection can be localized as a furuncle or boil or can involve the entire canal. If the entire canal is involved, there is likely to be itching, foul-smelling discharge, and sometimes some loss of hearing as well as pain. A boil causes severe pain and, when it drains, a brief pus discharge.

Infection of the middle ear, called *acute otitis media,* can occur at any age but is particularly common in children under 3 years of age. The first complaint usually is severe and persistent earache. In a young child, there may be little or no pain but the child may pull at the ear. Hearing loss may occur. And in a young child, fever up to 105°F, nausea, vomiting, and diarrhea may be present.

WHAT TO DO:

For outer ear infection, apply heat to the ear. Dry heat helps relieve pain and, particularly in the case of a boil in the outer ear canal, speeds resolution.

Get medical help.

For a boil, along with other treatment, codeine may be needed for the pain.

When the entire outer ear canal is infected, an antibiotic solution and, often, a solution of a corticosteroid such as hydrocortisone can be used, with the corticosteroid helping to reduce swelling in the ear so the antibiotic can penetrate all through the canal.

For middle ear infection, antibiotic treatment is often needed to relieve symptoms, bring infection under control, and reduce the possibility of complications such as mastoid infection and damage to the hearing mechanism. Among other often-valuable measures the physician may use are nose drops containing an agent such as phenylephrine to improve drainage through the eustachian tube, which is a canal connecting the middle ear and throat. Ephedrine sulfate or a similar drug may be given by mouth, and if you are allergic, an antihistamine may also be prescribed for a week or so to improve eustachian tube function.

Edema (Swelling with Fluids)

Edema, which used to be called *dropsy* when it involved the whole body, means abnormal fluid retention in body tissues, producing swelling. It is not a disease in itself but sometimes may be a symptom of disease or injury. Also, it can come from causes unrelated to injury or illness.

Edema of the ankles and feet is quite common, especially among people on their feet a lot, and disappears with rest. Edema of the ankles can also stem from tightness around the legs (as from garters or rolled stockings) or constriction of the thighs (by tight underclothing). When edema is constriction-caused, it is only necessary to remove the constricting garment and avoid further use.

An excessive intake of salt may be responsible for edema of the ankles and feet, since salt tends to hold water in the body and gravity may see to it that excess fluid settles below. An allergic reaction—such as to a dye in socks or an ingredient in cosmetics—may sometimes lead to swelling. Women often experience slight edema before the menstrual period (see MENSTRUAL DIFFICULTIES).

Edema, however, can also be an indication of beginning heart, kidney, or liver disease. And repeated episodes of ankle or other swelling, or an episode that lasts more than a day or two, should be investigated by a physician.

Elbow, Tennis

This painful problem can affect not only tennis players but also housewives who iron frequently, carpenters, do-it-yourselfers who do much screwdriving, officials who shake hands a lot, and others who forcefully clench their fists for long periods.

Tennis elbow is also known as *lateral humeral epicondylitis* and sometimes has been referred to as *radiohumeral bursitis*. Its exact nature is not entirely clear, but it does involve inflammation of a wrist-moving muscle at the point where the muscle attaches to the outside of the humerus, which is the upper arm bone extending from elbow to shoulder.

The affliction produces pain that may radiate from the elbow to the outer side of the arm and forearm.

WHAT TO DO: In mild cases, avoidance of any movements that cause pain may lead to gradual improvement.

A four-inch strap worn tightly around the forearm near the elbow may help provide relief and, if worn during activity that produces trouble, may help prevent recurrences.

In more severe cases, one or more injections of a local anesthetic, procaine, followed by hydrocortisone may be effective.

If your tennis elbow does in fact come from tennis, you may want to take some tips from recent sports medicine studies.

They indicate that use of a steel or aluminum racket and of a two-handed rather than one-handed backhand stroke make for the best chance of avoiding tennis elbow.

Something else to discuss with your pro: You are probably hitting the ball wrong, possibly too late. It is amazing how quickly the pain can disappear when, with a smooth stroke, the ball is hit squarely and with proper timing. Possibly, too, your hand grip is too tight because the racket handle is too small, too large, or slippery.

Eye, Black

This is a bruise or contusion of tissue around the eye. As in other contusions, the skin is not penetrated but tiny blood vessels are broken and blood seeps under the skin, producing discoloration and swelling.

Cold compresses, if applied immediately, help to slow the bleeding under the skin and thus to minimize the swelling and discoloration. Later, warm wet towels or compresses should be applied in order to speed the absorption of the discoloring fluid.

Medical help is generally required only if the eye has been injured or the blow was severe enough to break a bone of the face.

Eye, Foreign Body in

Foreign bodies—everything from sand, dust, paint chips, and bits of wood to rust and metal particles—are often blown or rubbed into the eyes. Beyond a harmful irritating effect, there may be danger that they will scratch the surface or become embedded in the eye.

The eye *must not* be rubbed; that may cause scratching or embedding. And the foreign body must be removed.

WHAT TO DO: Wash hands thoroughly before examining the

eye. Never use a toothpick, match, or any kind of instrument to try to remove the object.

Pull down the lower lid. If the object is on the lid's inner surface, lift it gently with the corner of a clean handkerchief or paper tissue; don't use dry cotton.

If the object is not under the lower lid, have the patient look down and, grasping the lashes of the upper lid gently, pull the lid forward and down over the lower lid, giving tears a chance to move the object out. If that doesn't work, use a matchstick or similar object that has no sharp edge or point, placing it horizontally on top of the upper lid, positioned so you can gently pull upward on the lid and evert it (turn it inside out) against the stick. You may then be able to lift off the object with a clean handkerchief corner and replace the lid by pulling gently downward on the lashes.

If the object has not been found, use a good light, shining it from both the front and side, to check the cornea, the clear membrane covering the colored part of the eye. If the object is there, do not touch it. Instead, wash the eye gently with clean water. If the object does not come off, it may be embed-

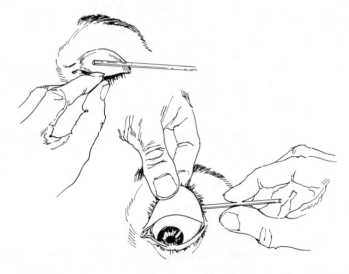

Fig. 14. Everting the upper eyelid to remove a foreign body.

ded. Apply a dry protective dressing as an eye patch and consult a physician or hospital emergency room.

If you succeed in removing an object but there is still a feeling that something is in the eye, the cornea may have been scraped or cut. If the corneal injury is minor, it will usually heal within 48 hours. Wash the eye out gently with water or a weak solution of boric acid.

A major corneal injury requires medical attention and so does a minor one, or what has seemed like a minor one, if symptoms persist beyond 48 hours.

If you have not found the foreign object, medical attention is needed. A physician can use a fluorescein stain and ultraviolet light, a slit lamp, or other measures to locate and remove the object or to identify and treat a laceration.

Eye Pain

Eye pain can be due to something as simple as a foreign body in the eye, which you may be able to remove readily (see EYE, FOREIGN BODY IN). Pain in the eye may also be referred there during a bout of sinusitis. It can also result from an injury or an acute infection of the eyelid, either or both of which may need medical attention.

But eye pain may have other causes which should be investigated by an ophthalmologist. These include *glaucoma* and *uveitis*. Uveitis is an inflammation of the uvea, which consists of the iris, ciliary body, and choroid of the eye, and is sometimes related to a specific allergy-causing agent but is often of unknown cause. Both glaucoma and uveitis are medically treatable—glaucoma often with eyedrops and uveitis with a corticosteroid such as prednisone.

Eye, Red (Conjunctivitis)

This is an inflammation of the mucous membrane, called the conjunctiva, which lines the eyelids and the white part of the eye. It can be caused by exposure to irritating chemicals, smoke, wind, dust, or intense light such as from an arc welder or a sunlamp. Commonly, it is caused by allergy and by bacterial and viral infections. And it may accompany the common cold and a childhood disease such as measles.

Generally, there is no risk of vision loss, but the viral and bacterial types are contagious, so it is wise to avoid contact with a person who has red eye and for that person to use his or her own towel.

When conjunctivitis is caused by a virus, it will usually clear in two or three days. When it is caused by bacteria, it may last longer but should clear on its own.

WHAT TO DO: Apply warm compresses to the eye several times a day.

Leave the eye unbandaged, unpatched, but sunglasses are helpful.

Aspirin can help ease distress.

Note this caution: Use no eye medication unless it has been prescribed by a physician. Drops or ointment containing a cortisone-like agent can cause serious damage if used in certain viral infections of the eye.

Note, too: If the redness lasts longer than three days and gives no indication of beginning to clear, an ophthalmologist should examine the eyes.

Also, there are certain signs that indicate when red eye may be extremely dangerous and an ophthalmologist should be seen without delay. These are

1. Blurring of vision or loss of some vision
2. Pain or a foreign body sensation when no foreign body is present in the eye
3. Discomfort from light (photophobia)

Blurring of vision in conjunctivitis may be due to the presence of mucus; if so, the blurring will clear with blinking. If blinking does not clear the vision, see an ophthalmologist immediately.

Eye, Spots in (Floaters)

Seeing spots (floaters) before one or both eyes is a frequent complaint among adults. Although such spots may seem alarming, very often they are innocuous.

Recently, when a Retina Foundation investigator checked eye physicians (ophthalmologists) present at a meeting in Boston, he found that 45 percent of them had the floaters, suggesting they are quite prevalent.

Commonly, they are little opaque bits of tissue debris floating in the vitreous humor, the transparent substance filling the part of the eyeball between the lens and retina. They are more common in highly nearsighted people and in older persons but tend to become less noticeable with time.

Since they sometimes can be associated with disease of the retina, it's advisable for anyone who has them to be checked by an ophthalmologist, not as an emergency matter but as a good precaution, and one that is likely to relieve anxiety.

If examination of the retina and vitreous shows no disease, there is no need for concern. In the relatively few cases in which the floaters are large and reduce vision seriously, surgery can be performed. It involves use of a needlelike instrument to break up and suck out the vitreous and replace it with a clear solution.

Eyelid Cyst or Tumor (Chalazion)

Caused by an infection of a sebaceous or oil gland of the eyelid, a chalazion is a painless, slow-growing cyst or tumor on the eyelid.

To begin with, it may resemble a sty, causing some lid swelling and irritation. After a few days, however, it stops looking stylike and becomes a painless, slowly growing, round mass.

Hot compresses help. A physician will also usually prescribe an ointment containing an antibiotic.

Chalazions usually disappear after a few months, but if one has not begun to do so after about six weeks, a physician can make an incision and clean it out.

Eyelid Swelling (Edema)

Edema, or fluid congestion, of one or both eyelids is commonly the result of allergy—often to eyedrop medication (such as atropine or epinephrine), other drugs, or cosmetics. Allergic reactions around the lids are frequently due to nail polish as a result of touching or scratching the lid with the fingers. Rarely, the congestion may be associated with trichinosis, the infection caused by a roundworm which enters the body in infected pork eaten when insufficiently cooked.

Often, the only treatment needed is to remove the allergy-producing material. Compresses of cold water over the closed lids are helpful in speeding reduction of edema and swelling.

If the swelling persists more than 24 hours, your physician can prescribe a medication containing a corticosteroid drug, such as 0.1 percent triamcinolone.

Faintness and Fainting

Fainting, in which consciousness is suddenly lost, usually results from an insufficient supply of blood to the brain. It may occur as a reaction to fear, hunger, pain, or any emotional or physical shock.

Prior to a faint, there usually are warning signs and symptoms: extreme pallor, sweating, coldness of the skin, light-headedness or dizziness, nausea.

WHAT TO DO: To prevent a fainting attack, anyone experiencing any of the warning indications should lie down if a bed is available, with legs somewhat elevated and collar and clothing loosened. Alternatively, sit down and lower the head between the knees for about five minutes. This will increase flow of blood and oxygen to the brain.

Once a faint has occurred, the victim should be left lying down, placed on his back, with legs elevated. Loosen any constricting clothing. If the faint has occurred indoors, open a window. Do not give any liquid unless the victim has revived. Do not pour water over the face because of the possibility that some may be sucked into the lungs. Bathe the face gently with cool water. If aromatic spirits of ammonia or smelling salts are available, hold them under the nose.

In several minutes, consciousness usually will be regained. Keep the victim lying down for another ten minutes, then have him get up slowly.

If recovery is not prompt, the problem could be more than a simple fainting spell and medical help is needed.

Note: Unfortunately, fainting has on occasion been mistaken for a heart attack and cardiopulmonary resuscitation (CPR) has been started when it was not needed. CPR is not entirely innocuous; it can produce injury; when needed, it can mean the difference between life and death; but its needless use may sometimes be tragic.

Remember

Remember these facts about fainting or "feeling faint" and you will be better able to handle the situation:

DIAGNOSIS:

1. The victim is usually well and without previous complaint (no pain, nausea, headache, etc.) but suddenly pales and loses consciousness.
2. The pulse is thready, feeble, or not detectable.
3. Breathing continues; signs of recovery occur quickly.

TREATMENT:

1. Have victim lie flat and elevate legs.
2. Loosen clothing.
3. Hold aromatic spirits of ammonia or smelling salts under nose.

DO NOT:

1. Give cardiopulmonary resuscitation (CPR).
2. Give any liquid by mouth.
3. Attempt to have victim sit up or rise.

Fever

One remarkable fact about fever is how almost anyone can sense its presence, even when the temperature elevation is only moderate. It is also a fact that fever accompanies a wide range of illnesses. And it is no less a fact that many people worry unduly about a temperature elevation that may even be normal for them. I know of one person who was deeply concerned when he forgot to take his thermometer along with him on a vacation.

Despite marked changes in air temperature, body temperature remains remarkably constant, within a range of about 1° or 1.5° Fahrenheit. Temperature control is achieved not only through the clothes you select but also by automatic dilation and constriction of blood vessels that carry blood to the skin and extremities—and by sweating which cools and shivering which increases muscle activity in order to generate more heat.

You should know that there is nothing sacrosanct about a so-called normal temperature of 98.6°F. Many people have normal temperatures in the range of 97° to 100°. Whatever the normal for an individual, almost certainly temperature will be lowest in the early morning, will rise during the day and usually reach a peak in the early evening.

Taking a temperature is simple enough. But you should know that there will be a difference between oral and rectal temperature. Rectal is usually half a degree to a whole degree higher because the thermometer tip gets closer to the central core of the body. Oral temperature is an adequate measure if the mouth is kept tightly closed while it is being taken— something difficult in children and adults who breathe through the mouth.

There is usually no need to worry about a temperature that does not exceed 100°F. Nor is there if the temperature is low unless it falls below 96°, in which case take the temperature again. If it still comes to less than 96°, better check to make certain that the thermometer is not broken.

Some more useful facts about fever: Your pulse rate will usually increase by about 10 beats a minute above your usual pulse rate with each degree of temperature elevation. If you should have fever associated with an infection, which is common, and your pulse rate does not go up, the likelihood is that you have a viral rather than bacterial infection.

Such uncomfortable symptoms as headache and chills,

which may be associated with fever, usually vary in intensity. So does temperature level. Except mostly in some chronic diseases of long standing, fever rarely stays at a constant high level but goes up and down.

It's the variation in temperature that is associated with some uncomfortable symptoms, such as chills followed by flushing as temperature rises and profuse sweating as the temperature falls.

CAUSES: Almost any illness can cause fever. Any injury to the body may do so. Most often, fever is associated with infection, bacterial or viral. Usually, when fever comes on abruptly and there are also headache, respiratory symptoms or gastrointestinal upset or both, malaise, and muscle and joint pains, the cause is viral.

WHAT TO DO: Even now, there is some uncertainty and controversy among physicians about the advisability of treating or letting alone a mild fever—say, up to about 102°. There is some evidence that temperature elevation may be part of the body's defense mechanism against infections.

If temperature climbs higher, however, it should be lowered or it can be debilitating. In a child under 3 years of age, it is usually advisable to avoid letting fever go beyond 103°, for there is some possibility of convulsions (a reassuring observation from recent studies is that such convulsions rarely have lasting effects). And certainly, in older children and adults, if confusion or delirium is associated with high fever, the fever should be treated promptly.

Usually, aspirin is the drug of choice, although acetaminophen can be used instead. In addition, when temperature is very high, sponging with cool water or rubbing alcohol will help. Sponge the entire body, paying particular attention to the armpits and between the legs.

Note that when aspirin or acetaminophen is used, there will be temporary relief of associated symptoms, but there may also be some discomfort as the drug brings the temperature down and then the temperature climbs again. For more comfort, aspirin or acetaminophen can be taken about every four hours. Be careful, though, since the fever provides some indication of the severity of the underlying problem, and keeping temperature down constantly with drugs may mask increasing severity of an illness.

Fluid loss with fever can be substantial even if there is no apparent sweating. So fluids should be given. Water can be used. Water, however, will not replace the vital chemicals lost in perspiration—and for their replacement, the old-fashioned idea of chicken soup has merit.

Obviously, the best treatment for fever is treatment of the cause if that is possible. With a viral illness such as flu, there is no curative drug, and home treatment (see INFLUENZA) is justified unless complications develop.

It can be especially important, if a child is the patient, to get in touch with the physician if the child has a stiff neck, rash, breathing difficulty, looks very ill, or is lethargic.

Fever Blisters (Cold Sores)

These itching or stinging sores on the skin or mucous membranes, known both as fever blisters and as cold sores, usually occur with a cold or fever, and are caused by a virus, herpes simplex. They may also follow exposure to sun and wind, a gastrointestinal upset, or even emotional distress.

They usually dry up after several days, form a crust, and clear within a week or so. Drying lotions or liquids such as calamine, camphor spirit, or 70 percent alcohol may be helpful, and can be applied with bits of cotton. During the onset period, cold cream may provide some relief. When the crust has formed, zinc oxide applied to it may speed recovery.

Fever, Scarlet (See CHILDHOOD DISEASES, COMMUNICABLE)

Fibromyositis (See MUSCLE AND JOINT PAIN, TENDERNESS, STIFFNESS)

Fingernail Injury

When the tip of a finger is hurt—as, for example, when it is slammed in a door—the fingernail is likely to become black and blue, and there may be intense throbbing pain in the fingertip.

The crushing leads to bleeding under the nail, and a little blood collection (hematoma) may form, pushing on nail and bone and causing the pain.

WHAT TO DO: Apply cold compresses immediately.

If pain increases over the next several hours, it may be necessary to drill the nail to get the blood out. If done properly, the drilling produces no pain and is a simple procedure. The nail itself has no pain sensitivity.

It is wise to go to an emergency room for the drilling, since when done by an expert it takes just a few seconds. It is also best done under sterile conditions.

If, however, such a facility is not available, you can easily treat the condition yourself.

Fig. 15. Drilling hole in fingernail with pocket knife.

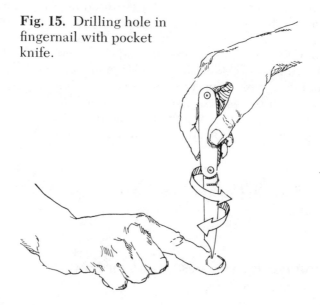

An ordinary pocketknife can be used. Sharpen its tip. Heat the tip over a flame or dip it into boiling water for a few minutes to sterilize it. Be sure to let it cool before using it, but make certain it touches no other object or surface before being used.

Have someone help you by holding the finger, so it does not move, on a firm flat surface such as a table. The knife tip then can be placed at the center of the discolored area of the nail near the cuticle and gently turned in a back and forth drilling motion.

When a hole is through the nail, a small drop of blood will appear. At that point, drill no deeper or you will touch the nail bed, which is tender, and there may be some likelihood as well of causing infection.

Apply a gauze dressing or a clean handkerchief to absorb the blood. Pain relief is likely to follow very quickly.

To continue the absorption of blood and protect the nail, cover it for several days with a gauze Band-Aid or equivalent.

If drilling fails to provide relief, a physician should be consulted.

A physician should also be consulted if there is a bony deformity, which may indicate a dislocation or fracture. If the fingertip hangs down and cannot be straightened, there may be a torn tendon that will need surgical repair.

Finger Pain, Numbness, Tingling

These sensations can be due to prolonged pressure on a nerve or compression of an artery, which cuts off blood supply. For example, resting the wrist against a hard object, particularly falling asleep with the wrist in such a position, can produce finger pain, numbness, and tingling.

Another cause is a condition known as the *carpal tunnel syndrome*. The median nerve, a major nerve of the hand, passes through the wrist in a tunnel under the carpal ligament. Compression of this nerve can lead to finger pain, numbness, and tingling.

The carpal tunnel syndrome, which is most common in middle-aged women, may result from excessive wrist movement, arthritis, swelling of the wrist, or overgrowth of bone and connective tissue. A tight wristwatch band may sometimes be an offender.

WHAT TO DO: Conservative treatment may be effective for the carpal tunnel syndrome. This means resting the wrist, using a splint to give the irritated median nerve a chance to heal. Several weeks may be needed.

In severe chronic cases, rapid cure can be achieved with surgery in which the tunnel is opened and the carpal ligament is divided, ending the nerve compression.

Fishhook Accidents

Penetration of the skin by a fishhook is no rare accident. If the hook has penetrated only a little way—up to the barb or only slightly past it—it often can be backed out readily.

If the hook has penetrated deeper and the barb has become embedded, it is best, if possible, to have a physician remove it.

If medical aid is not available, the best method of removal may be to push the hook on through until the barb protrudes, then snip the hook either at the barb or at the shank and remove.

After either of these maneuvers, if there has been very little bleeding, encourage some temporary blood flow as a help in eliminating any infectious organisms by gentle pressure on the wound. Don't squeeze hard. Then apply a protective sterile dressing and get medical attention as soon as possible.

If the hook is large and has produced considerable damage, or if it is in a critical area about the face or eye, it is best not to try to remove it. Cover the wound and hook with a sterile dressing and get the victim to a doctor.

Fit (See CONVULSION)

Flatulence (Gas)

Some gas in the gastrointestinal tract is normal. A certain amount is there because air is swallowed with food and drink; some gas is released by food ingredients and some is formed

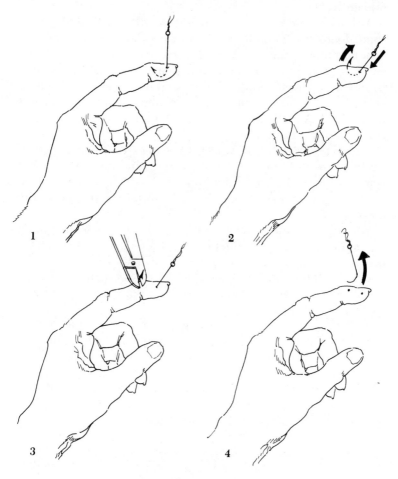

Fig. 16. Removing a fishhook.

by bacterial fermentation in the intestines; and some gas even diffuses into the intestines from blood.

But excessive gas is a very common and often painful complaint.

If you are a chronic victim of gas discomfort, it could well be because you swallow excessive amounts of air and are among the large group of people who are aerophagics (see AIR SWALLOWING), and attention to correcting this could help significantly.

Although no one food is a culprit for all people at all times, some foods are notable for their gas-producing tendencies. Among them: onions, raw apples, radishes, baked beans, cucumbers, milk, melon, cauliflower, chocolate, coffee, lettuce, peanuts, and eggs. Additionally, souffles, beaten omelettes, cake, fresh bread, and meringues contain more gas than do other foods. And effervescent drinks and malteds may contribute a significant amount.

WHAT TO DO FOR AN ACUTE EPISODE OF FLATULENCE: If you're suffering from a bout of gas pain and distention, a hot water bottle or heating pad applied to the abdomen and some gentle massage may help. So may a pint-sized, lukewarm, tap-water enema.

You can also often speed up elimination of gas by assuming a position such as the "telephoning teen-ager" posture. This involves lying stomach down on a bed, with legs bent at the knees at a 90-degree angle, and with arms bent at the elbows and turned toward each other and stretched out ahead and supporting the head.

As for commercial gas-relieving preparations, some contain simethicone, a silicone material that theoretically should— and sometimes does—help by stimulating release of entrapped gas.

Plain charcoal tablets are often helpful but are not always readily available, and you may have to insist that your pharmacist make some effort to order them for you.

Note: A first acute episode of abdominal distention, with the abdomen becoming increasingly blown up and inability to pass gas at the rectum, can mean intestinal obstruction. This is an emergency calling for immediate medical help and possibly surgery.

Floaters (See EYE, SPOTS IN)

Flu (See INFLUENZA)

Food Allergies (See ALLERGIES)

Food Infection (See GASTROENTERITIS, ACUTE)

Food Poisoning (See GASTROENTERITIS, ACUTE)

Foreign Object in the Nose

Whatever the object may be, calm the patient. Try to withdraw the object. If it does not come out readily, don't try any further. Excessive probing may shove the object in deeper and cause injury to the nostril. Don't allow violent nose blowing. Let a physician get the object out.

Foreign Object in the Skin

Many types of objects can penetrate the skin and become embedded. They include wood splinters, glass fragments, metal chips, pieces of pencil lead, thorns, buckshot. (See also FISHHOOK ACCIDENTS.)

Often these objects remain in the skin tissues or in the tissues just below.

WHAT TO DO: Clean the area with soap and water.

If the object is in the surface tissue, use tweezers, sterilized over a flame, or in boiling water, to pull it out. If the object is embedded just below the skin, use the tip of a needle sterilized in a flame or boiling water to lift it out or, if necessary, to slightly enlarge the puncture hole to make extraction with either the needle or sterilized tweezers easier. Any object that has become deeply embedded, no matter how small or large, is best left for a physician to remove.

Once the object has been removed, wash thoroughly with soap and water around the puncture site and apply a Band-Aid or, if necessary, a bandage.

If you think there is any likelihood of infection developing, warm soaks for half an hour at a time, one to three times a day, for several days can be used. Check with your physician, too, about possible need for tetanus immunization or tetanus toxoid booster injection.

If an infection should develop—manifested by swelling and redness, throbbing pain, tenderness, fever, pus beneath the skin or draining out, swollen glands—see a physician for treatment. If there is any delay, remain quiet, elevate the area if possible, and apply warm, moist cloths or towels as a temporary expedient.

Foreign Objects, Swallowed

Children manage to swallow an incredible variety of nonfood items. If you're confronted with the problem, don't panic.

Is the object small and round—for example, beads, button, coin, marble? Such objects usually make their way, without difficulty and without causing any distress, through the gastrointestinal tract and are duly eliminated. You don't have to give cathartics or change the diet. If there is pain, of course consult your physician. Otherwise, keep a careful lookout for several days at stools to make certain the object is eliminated.

Some objects do carry risk—straight pins or open safety pins, bones, bobby pins, other sharp or straight items. If such an object has been swallowed, it can be located by a physician by x-ray and removed with special instruments.

If an object should lodge in the throat and cut off breathing, the condition is an emergency for which the Heimlich maneuver should be used without delay (see CHOKING ON FOOD AND OTHER OBJECTS, p. 40).

If the object has entered the windpipe or the tubes leading to the lung, you will recognize this by the coughing that occurs. This situation calls for x-ray to locate the object and its removal by a specialist in endoscopy. *Most important:* Keep the child *sitting* or *standing.* Do *not* bend him forward or slap the back. Bending forward can cause the object to fall against the vocal cords, closing off the small slitlike space between them, causing strangulation. Back slapping can drive the object deeper.

Fractures, Dislocations, Sprains, and Strains

There is sometimes confusion about definitions. To clarify:

A *fracture* is a break or crack in a bone. A closed or simple fracture is one in which bone does not cut through the skin. An open or compound fracture is one in which broken ends of bone protrude through the skin.

A *dislocation* is a separation or displacement of the end of a bone from a joint such as at the shoulder, elbow, finger, or thumb.

A *sprain* is an injury to the soft tissue about a joint. Muscles, ligaments, and tendons, which are attached to bones, serve both to move them and to hold them in place. In a sprain, the muscles, ligaments, and tendons—and blood vessels as well —are stretched or torn. The most common sprains are of the ankles, fingers, wrists, and knees.

A *strain* is a muscle injury in which muscle fibers are stretched and sometimes partially torn. A common strain is of the back due to improper lifting using the back instead of the legs.

Fractures

Bone fractures most commonly result from falls, automobile accidents, and injuries during sports and recreational activities. Sometimes, in an older person, because of bone brittleness, a break may result from only relatively slight injury.

RECOGNIZING FRACTURES: Some are obvious. The victim may hear or feel a bone snap or may be aware of broken bones rubbing together and producing a grating sensation. There may be a difference in shape or length of a bone on one side of the body in comparison with its counterpart on the other side. Or there may be an obvious deformity. Other indications of fracture include swelling, discoloration, and pain or tenderness to touch.

Often, however, not enough clear-cut indications are present to be certain that the problem is a fracture as opposed to a sprain. An x-ray is needed to be certain. Whenever there is any doubt, treat for fracture.

WHAT TO DO: Don't try to set a fracture yourself. Your objectives should be to prevent further injury, keep broken bone ends and nearby joints from moving, and look for and treat shock (see SHOCK, p. 28) if it is present.

Keep the victim warm. Apply an ice bag to the painful area to help decrease swelling and inflammation.

If a broken bone protrudes through the skin and there is bleeding, cut away clothing if necessary and place a pad—sterile compress or clean handkerchief or cloth—over the wound and press firmly directly over the wound. Do not wash or probe the wound. If a bone fragment protrudes, cover the wound with a large sterile bandage or a freshly laundered towel or sheet.

If the victim must be moved in order to receive medical attention, immobilize the fracture with splints to prevent further injury.

For *splinting* you can use anything that will keep the fractured bone from moving. That includes rolled-up newspapers or magazines, boards, straight sticks, umbrella.

Make splints long enough to extend past the joints both above and below the break. Pad the splints with whatever is available—clean rags, cotton, or anything soft. Tie in place snugly but not too tightly with bandages, belts, neckties, or strips of clothing. If an arm is splinted, check the pulse at the wrist and inspect fingers often for swelling or blueness, an indication that tying has been too tight. If the victim complains of numbness, tingling, or inability to move fingers or toes, loosen ties immediately.

Don't try to straighten a broken arm or leg. Splint simply to immobilize the break, and leave bone setting to a physician.

COLLARBONE FRACTURE: Severe pain and swelling may occur at the site of the break, which sometimes can be found by gently running fingers over the area. The shoulder on the injured side will often be lower than the other, since the collarbone is needed to support the shoulder. Put the arm on the injured side in a sling. Adjust the sling so the hand is slightly above level of the elbow. Tie the arm to the side of the body with a triangular, roller or other bandage—snugly but not so tight as to interfere with circulation. You should be able to feel the pulse at the wrist after the bandage is in place. If not, either the bandage is too tight or the elbow is bent at too acute an angle.

SHOULDER BLADE (SCAPULA) FRACTURE: Place the forearm on the injured side in a sling so it is held across the chest horizontally. Then bandage the upper arm to the chest wall.

UPPER ARM (HUMERUS) FRACTURE: Apply a splint and tie in place above and below the break. Place a pad in the armpit, and support the forearm with a sling, making certain the forearm is positioned so there is no upward pressure at the site of the break. Bandage the upper arm to the chest wall.

ELBOW FRACTURE: An elbow fracture may involve the lower part of the humerus (of the upper arm) or bones of the forearm. Do not attempt to move the arm at the elbow joint if you suspect a fracture. If the arm is either bent or straight, let it remain that way.

If the arm is straight, apply a well-padded splint extending from fingertips to armpit along both sides of the arm and secure with ties. Do not allow the splint to press into the armpit or it will interfere with blood circulation.

If the arm is bent, put it in a sling and bind it firmly to the side of the body.

FOREARM OR WRIST FRACTURE: Apply well-padded splints

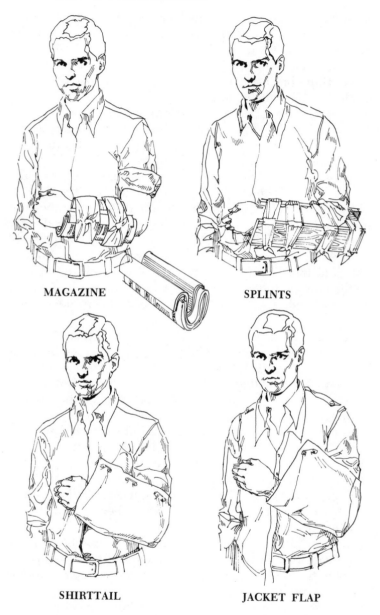

MAGAZINE   SPLINTS

SHIRTTAIL   JACKET   FLAP

Fig. 17. TOP: Splinting a forearm. BOTTOM: Jacket flap.

on each side from hand to elbow. Support the arm in a sling adjusted so the fingers are about four inches higher than the elbow (or a little less in a child). Leave fingertips uncovered so you can watch for any swelling or blueness; if either or both appear, carefully loosen the splint or sling slightly. If a doctor cannot be reached, at night remove the sling and allow the arm to rest on a pillow with hand higher than elbow.

FINGER FRACTURE: Immobilize the injured finger with a splint. Use a sling to support the hand. Keep the hand higher than the elbow, day and night.

UPPER LEG FRACTURE: With fracture of the femur, or upper leg bone, there is usually severe pain and disability. The foot usually is turned outward, and the limb is shortened because muscular spasm causes overlapping of bone ends. Watch for

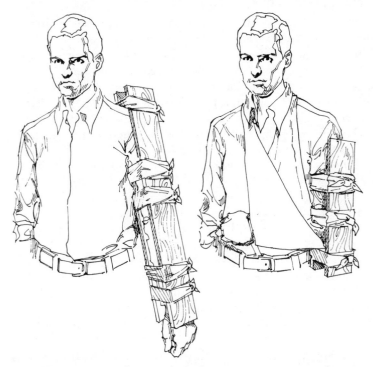

Fig. 18. LEFT: Splinting whole arm. RIGHT: Splinting upper arm.

and treat shock if it appears (see p. 28). If the victim will be moved only a short distance on a stretcher, put a blanket between the legs, then bind the legs together. In this way, the uninjured leg acts as a splint. If it is necessary to use splints, pad them well. One splint should reach, on the outer side, from just below the armpit to below the heel; the other, on the inner side, should extend from just below the groin to below the heel.

KNEECAP FRACTURE: The kneecap, or *patella*, a small bone just in front of the knee joint, plays an important role in knee joint motion. When the patella is fractured, the pull of large leg muscles tends to separate broken fragments. Look for pain and tenderness at the fracture site, and inability to straighten out the leg. Sometimes, by gently running fingers over the kneecap, you will find a groove due to separation of the bony fragments. Gently straighten out the leg. The best splint is a board, four to six inches wide, long enough to reach from buttock to just below the heel. Pad well with clean rags or other material. Tie limb to board, leaving the kneecap itself exposed, since there may be rapid swelling. Check every 20 minutes or so to see that bindings do not cut off circulation. Loosen slightly if necessary. If no board is available, place a pillow or rolled-up blanket under the knee and tie in place. Transport the victim lying down.

LOWER LEG FRACTURE: Lower leg bones are the shinbone, or tibia, which carries body weight, and the fibula on the outer side of the leg, which forms the outer wall of the ankle. Apply well-padded splints on both sides of leg and foot, extending from just below buttock and groin to below heel. Keep foot pointing upward. Check frequently to make sure circulation to lower leg and foot is not cut off. If splints are not available, place blanket or towels between legs and tie legs together.

ANKLE AND FOOT FRACTURE: Remove shoe and sock quickly, since swelling may be rapid. Cut off shoe and sock if necessary rather than cause further injury by pulling off. If there is an open wound, apply bulky sterile dressings if possible. Apply blanket or small pillow as a splint from several inches above the ankle to beyond the toes. Bandage in place snugly, with one tie running under the foot, another about the

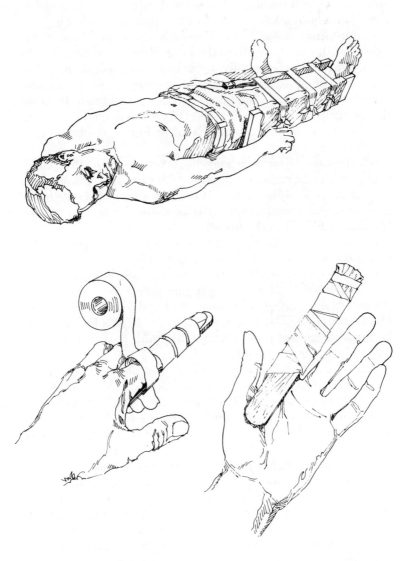

Fig. 19. TOP: Splint for leg. BOTTOM: Finger splint.

ankle, and the third above the second. Leave toes exposed to check circulation. Keep foot on pillow higher than knee.

PELVIC FRACTURE: The pelvis—a basin-shaped bony structure extending outward from the base of the spine and curving toward the front of the body—provides a connection between spine and legs. It also protects many important organs and blood vessels lying in the lower part of the abdomen. Because these organs and vessels may be seriously damaged by broken bone ends, a pelvic fracture is a grave injury, requiring very careful handling.

A symptom of fracture may be severe pain in the pelvic region while standing or walking; the pain may diminish or disappear while lying down. If there has been damage to organs or blood vessels, there may be difficulty in urinating or blood may appear in the urine.

If you're not certain but have any reason to suspect a fracture after an injury to the pelvic region, treat as a fracture.

Combat shock, which may be severe (see SHOCK, p. 28). Bandage knees and ankles together. Keep the victim lying down. He will probably be most comfortable on his back with knees straight, but let him keep his knees bent if he wishes. If he must be moved to receive medical aid, transport on back on rigid stretcher or board.

RIB FRACTURE: There is usually pain at the point of the break. Breathing is shallow since taking a deep breath or coughing increases pain. The point of fracture sometimes can be felt by running fingers gently along the rib. If the lung has been damaged by a broken rib, frothy or bright red blood may be coughed up.

If the broken rib has penetrated the skin and air is blowing in and out of the wound or just sucking into it, apply an airtight dressing. The dressing should be held firmly in place with adhesive tape and your hand. The important thing is to keep air from getting into the wound, since it will collapse the lung. Get the victim to lie quietly. If he must be moved to a doctor, move him lying down.

If the chest is not punctured, bandage firmly to restrict rib motion. To do so, first loosely tie a triangular bandage or other broad bandage around the body at chest level so the knot will

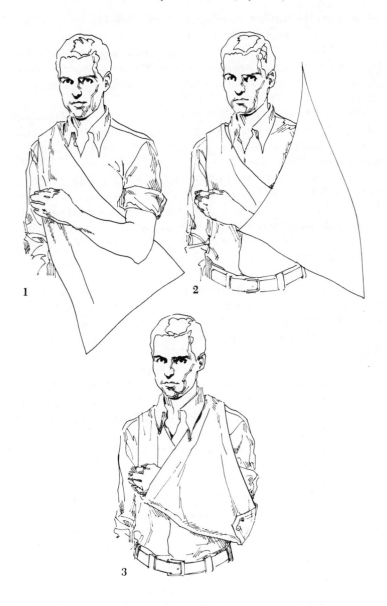

Fig. 20. Applying a triangular bandage.

be on the side opposite the break. Put a folded cloth under the knot. As the victim breathes out, tighten the bandage and tie snugly, but not so tight as to restrict breathing too much. Repeat with two or more bandages in the same way so they overlap slightly and cover the site of the fracture and adjacent areas.

NOSE FRACTURE: Look for pain and tenderness in and about the nose, swelling and discoloration, possibly a change in the usual shape of the nose. If there is bleeding, hold the lower end of the nose between thumb and index finger and firmly press the sides of the nose against the middle partition (septum) for four or five minutes. Release pressure gradually. Apply cold cloths over the nose. Have the victim sit up, hold head back slightly, and breathe through the mouth. Do not splint. If there is a wound on the nose, apply a compress or protective dressing and fix in place with adhesive tape or bandage. Get to a doctor as soon as possible.

JAW FRACTURE: Look for pain on movement and inability to close the jaw properly. Teeth do not line up correctly. There is difficulty in speaking, drinking, swallowing. Raise the jaw gently with the palm of your hand to bring lower and upper teeth together. Put a bandage under the chin and tie the ends over the top of the head to support the jaw. Remove the bandage immediately if the victim starts to vomit. Support the jaw with your hand. Rebandage when vomiting stops. If medical help is not available for several days, nourishment can be taken through a straw.

NECK OR BACK FRACTURE: If the victim is not readily able to open and close his fingers or if there is numbness or tingling around his shoulders, the neck may be broken. If his fingers work but he cannot move his feet or toes, or if he has tingling or numbness in the legs or pain when he tries to move the back or neck, his back may be broken. If the victim is unconscious and you suspect spinal injury, treat as if the neck were fractured.

Loosen clothing around neck and waist. Cover with blankets. Don't allow the victim to move his head. Don't lift his head even to give him water. Any movement may cause paralysis. Watch his breathing and be ready to start resuscitation if necessary (p. 49).

Get a doctor or ambulance. The victim should not be moved unless there is no chance of getting medical help at the scene. If a move must be made, it must be done with *extreme caution*. A twist or bend of broken neck or spine can paralyze or kill. Take extreme care to avoid moving the neck or spine while loading the victim onto a rigid stretcher or board. Pad the head well at the sides to prevent motion. Tie hands across chest and tie head and body rigidly to the board. Pad under the neck.

SKULL FRACTURE: Chief reason for concern in skull fracture is not so much the bone itself as the tissues beneath it. Brain injury or concussion can occur whether there has been an actual fracture or not.

Look for a bump or cut at the site of injury. The victim may be unconscious, or dazed and mentally confused. There may be bleeding or drainage of clear watery fluid from ears, mouth, nose. Pupils of the eyes may be different in size.

Keep the victim lying down. Prop up his head and shoulders if his face is either normal in color or flushed. Lower his head slightly if his face is pale. If a move is necessary, move the victim in lying-down position. Apply sterile gauze and bandage to an open scalp wound. Get a doctor as soon as possible but don't leave the victim alone. Keep alert. Be ready, if the victim should start choking on blood, to lower his head and turn it carefully to the side to drain the mouth. Wipe out the blood from the mouth with a clean handkerchief if necessary.

Dislocations

In a dislocation, the end of a bone is displaced from its normal position in a joint. The surrounding ligaments may suffer some injury. A dislocation may result from a fall, blow against a joint, sudden twisting of the joint, or sudden muscle contraction. Most often affected are fingers, thumb, shoulder, or elbow.

Symptoms may include swelling, obvious deformity, pain upon motion, tenderness to touch, discoloration.

Putting a serious dislocation back into place (i.e., "reducing" it) is a physician's job. Unless properly relocated and cared for, there may be repeated dislocation and disability. All dislocations should be handled in much the same way as fractures.

Keep the dislocated part quiet. Don't try to reduce it. Splint and immobilize the joint in the dislocated position. Apply cold compresses. Seek medical attention promptly.

Support a dislocated elbow or shoulder in a loose sling so it is kept immobilized during transport. If a hip is dislocated, move the victim on a wide board or stretcher made rigid. Use a pad of blankets or clothing large enough to support the leg on the injured side in the position the victim holds it.

Sometimes, in the case of a dislocated finger, when medical attention will be long delayed, gentle traction may be tried. Pull cautiously—very cautiously—on the finger to try to bring the bone into place. If unsuccessful, do not persist. And do not attempt this on a dislocated thumb, since there are more difficulties in the way and more risk of added injury.

One of the most common ski injuries is thumb dislocation. It results from grasping the top of the pole and ski strap between thumb and index finger. The slightest fall puts tremendous twisting force on the base of the thumb, pushing it out of its socket. To avoid this injury, either put your hand downward through the loop of the strap and grasp only the pole, with the loop lying loosely around the wrist—or, better still, use a strapless pole or a strap that detaches automatically from the pole under pressure.

Sprains

Sprains, as noted previously, are injuries to soft tissues surrounding joints, with stretching and sometimes tearing or partial tearing of ligaments, muscles, tendons, and blood vessels. Ankles, fingers, wrists, and knees are most commonly affected.

Symptoms include swelling, tenderness, pain on motion, and sometimes discoloration of skin over a large area because of rupture of small blood vessels.

It is often difficult even for a physician to tell a sprain from a fracture without an x-ray. If the sprain seems severe, or if you have any reason to suspect a fracture, splint the part and treat as you would a fracture.

Otherwise, rest and elevate the injured part. If ankle or knee is affected, there should be no walking. Loosen or remove shoes. Swelling, because it can cut off circulation, may sometimes cause more trouble than the original sprain. To minimize swelling, elevate the leg and apply cold compresses. Cold helps contract blood vessels, minimize leakage of blood, tends to reduce swelling and pain. For wrist sprain, put the arm in a sling adjusted so the fingers are about four inches higher than the elbow. For elbow sprain, also put the arm in a sling. Apply cold compresses.

In mild sprains, keep the injured part immobilized and raised for at least 24 hours, continuing the cold applications.

If swelling and pain persist, get medical help.

Strains

Strains are muscle injuries due to overexertion, with muscle fibers stretched, sometimes partially torn. While strains can occur in any muscle, most frequent are those of back muscles, usually caused by lifting.

Symptoms include sharp pain or cramp at the time of injury; stiffness and pain on movement, which may increase within a few hours; and some swelling of the affected muscle.

Have the victim rest the injured area, sitting or lying quietly in a comfortable position. Apply hot compresses. Massage gently—in the direction of the heart, to stimulate blood flow in that direction. Gentle massage may help lessen stiffness. For a strained back, a bed board under the mattress helps by providing firm support. (See also BACK PAIN.)

Frostbite

If you're exposed to very low temperatures and reach shelter chilled to the bone with nipped fingers, toes, cheeks, nose or ears, what should you do?

Do *not* follow the ancient suggestion to rub the frostbitten parts with snow or ice. Recent studies have shown that immediate application of gentle warmth leaves you with less tissue damage and less likelihood of infection or gangrene.

In frostbite, ice crystals may form in or between cells either superficially or in the underlying skin tissues. Usually, the frostbitten area is small, and the most common sites are nose, cheeks, ears, fingers, and toes.

With frostbite, the skin changes to a whitish or grayish-yellow appearance. Sometimes, early on, pain may be felt; later, the area feels very cold, hard, and numb.

WHAT TO DO: Get into a warm room as soon as possible. Rapidly rewarm the frostbitten areas. The best way, if possible, is a warm, not hot, bath. Hot drinks to warm the whole body from within are important helps, and this is one instance where the alcoholic drink to stimulate the circulation is called for.

If a bath is not possible, wrap in warm blankets.

Out in the field, snuggling next to a warm companion may be effective. So, too, may be rewarming the hands by placing them in the armpits or on the abdomen.

Vital note: Whatever method of warming you use, the temperature must not exceed 110° Fahrenheit or 43° Celsius because the affected areas are numb and susceptible to burns. If you use a bath and have a thermometer, keep the water temperature in the 100° to 110°F range, adding warm water as needed. If you have no thermometer, test water temperature by pouring some over the inner surface of your forearm. *Do not use* a heat lamp or hot water bottle, or expose frostbitten areas to a hot stove.

And do not rub or massage: this may favor gangrene.

When the frostbitten area becomes flushed, stop rewarming.

Do *not* break any blisters.

Soon after rewarming, exercise the frostbitten part.

Take aspirin for pain.

Get medical help.

Gallbladder Disease

A common problem, mostly associated with gallstones, gallbladder disease is responsible each year for the hospitalization of about half a million people in the United States.

It can be mistaken for other conditions—*yet it is possible for you to suspect when you have a gallbladder problem.*

The gallbladder is a pear-shaped sac in the upper right part of the abdomen, under the liver, which stores bile coming from the liver. The three- to four-inch-long sac holds up to about two ounces of bile and releases it when food containing fat has been eaten and arrives in the intestine. The bile flows from the gallbladder through a passage called the *cystic duct* into the *common bile duct*, which arises in the liver. And from the common bile duct bile empties into the intestine to help in fat digestion.

The gallbladder is not essential; when it is removed, the liver can supply bile directly to the intestine through the common bile duct.

Trouble with the gallbladder usually involves stonelike masses, called *calculi* or *gallstones*. Their presence is known as *cholelithiasis*. Why they form is not definitively understood, but they tend to affect women more often than men, and there is evidence of a relationship with obesity.

Gallstones are peculiar. They are present in many people without ever once causing any difficulties. On the other hand, in many others they are associated with chronic inflammation of the gallbladder, producing episodes of discomfort, and they may also lead to very painful acute inflammation (*acute cholecystitis*).

RECOGNIZING A GALLBLADDER ATTACK: Chances are, if you suffer a severe gallbladder attack—an episode of acute cholecystitis—you will have had milder episodes before.

You may well have had bouts of what seemed like dyspepsia, or indigestion, with abdominal gas, belching, nausea, and pain in the upper abdomen—all made worse by large or fatty meals. Like many sufferers, you may have learned, even without realizing that gallbladder disease was involved, to avoid fatty and greasy foods.

At some point, however, may come the severe acute attack when a gallstone manages to work itself into a position where it plugs the bile outlet of the gallbladder into the cystic duct. When that happens—and it usually makes itself known at night or in the early morning—there will be pain in the right upper quadrant (or quarter) of the abdomen as the blocked gallbladder, distended with bile, tries to contract and squeeze out both the bile and the blocking stone. Commonly, too, nausea, vomiting, and flatulence are present.

The pain in the right upper quadrant may start suddenly or gradually. It may be aching at first but then becomes very severe. In addition, the pain commonly will radiate or spread to the back and right shoulder.

1, 2, 3 for diagnosis: You can suspect an acute cholecystitis attack on the basis of three indications:

1. Pain in the upper right quadrant, often accompanied by nausea, vomiting, and flatulence.
2. Radiation of the pain to the back and right shoulder.
3. If you press down, or have someone else do so, on the right upper quadrant of the abdomen, the area will be tender.

WHAT TO DO: You will need medical help.

Generally, an acute gallbladder attack does not require immediate emergency surgery as in the case of acute appendicitis. The reason is that the primary condition in the acute gallbladder attack is not infection as in appendicitis. There is also a possibility that the blocking stone may shake loose and float back into the gallbladder, freeing the outlet—or, in some instances, that it may even manage to pass through the cystic duct into the common bile duct and into the intestine to be eliminated.

Even so, because multiple stones are usually present and there is the likelihood of future attacks, surgical removal is usually advisable.

If the fact that you have had a gallbladder attack is proven beyond question by an x-ray of the organ showing the presence of gallstones, the surgeon may indicate he would like to operate immediately.

Although this can be acceptable treatment, it is safe in almost every instance (except as to be noted) to delay surgery, allowing the acute attack to subside, helped by diet and, if necessary, antibiotics. This will provide time for thorough examination and study to make certain no other problems are present which also should be treated.

After a few weeks, the gallbladder can be removed under better circumstances than as an emergency measure.

The operation, called *cholecystectomy*, removes the entire gallbladder with the stones it contains. The procedure, carried out under general anesthesia, usually takes about an hour. An incision is made below the ribs and to the right of the navel. The hospital stay may be as brief as eight days. In the hands of an experienced surgeon, the odds are better than 90 percent that the operation will be curative.

In the case of some older people and diabetics, however, it may be advisable not to delay surgery; or if there is to be a wait, they may require close watch in a hospital. Both are more likely than others to have a degree of artery hardening which may reduce blood circulation to the gallbladder as it does to other parts of the body. In such cases, there is some risk of necrosis, or gangrene, of portions of the wall of the gallbladder which can lead to perforation and leakage of bile into the abdominal (peritoneal) cavity, a serious emergency situation.

JAUNDICE (SKIN YELLOWING): A mild degree of yellowing of the skin may occur with any acute attack of gallbladder disease. But if the yellowness is deep, or deepens in a short period, it can mean that a gallstone has gotten out of the gallbladder into the common bile duct and become lodged there, blocking the flow of bile that would ordinarily empty into the intestine. The bile then backs up into the liver and is absorbed in the blood, producing deep skin yellowing.

Here again, emergency surgery is not essential unless there is some likelihood that the gallbladder is or may become gangrenous. Also, if the yellow color increases in intensity, surgery should be performed quickly. Otherwise, medical measures usually can help until the acute problem subsides, so the patient is in the best general condition for surgery. The operation removes the gallbladder (since it is the source of the stone), and the stone or stones are cleared out of the common duct so bile can flow freely again, as needed.

NEW DEVELOPMENTS: A recently developed instrument is

a *flexible fiberoptic endoscope*. A physician can pass it through the esophagus and stomach into the duodenum, the first portion of the small intestine. This can be done gently, with mild sedation, and without need for general anesthesia. It is then possible to thread a tube into the common bile duct, without open surgery, and perform x-rays, drain the duct, and remove stones in the duct by cutting the circular muscle that lies where the common bile duct enters the duodenum. This procedure must be carried out by a trained specialist. It is available in many large hospitals now.

Another new development that may substantially reduce the number of gallbladder operations is the use of medication which, over a period of time, can dissolve certain types of gallstones. It is under long-term—and thus far promising—trial at several medical centers.

Gas (See FLATULENCE)

Gastritis, Acute

Sudden, sometimes violent in onset, and usually lasting only briefly, this is a common disorder—an inflammation of the mucous membrane lining of the stomach.

It may be the result of acute alcoholism, drugs such as aspirin, hot spicy foods, foods (notably milk, eggs, fish) to which an individual may be allergic, bacteria or toxins in food poisoning, or an acute viral illness.

Symptoms may include nausea, vomiting, headache, dizziness, sensations of fullness, loss of appetite, general malaise.

Another form of gastritis, *acute corrosive gastritis*, may be caused by swallowing strong acids or alkalis, iodine, potassium permanganate, or other corrosive materials.

In acute corrosive gastritis, symptoms and signs will depend upon the kind and amount of corrosive material swallowed. The lips, tongue, mouth, and throat may be corroded; usually the esophagus, or gullet, is inflamed and painful and there is difficulty in swallowing. Often the abdomen is tender and rigid; blood may be vomited and may appear in stools; the pulse may race.

WHAT TO DO: For acute corrosive gastritis, immediate hospitalization is needed. The corrosive agent must be removed by stomach tube or emetic drugs or be neutralized by antidotes. Transfusion of blood or plasma may be needed. And a drug such as meperidine may be required for severe pain.

Fortunately the mucous membrane lining of the stomach is replaced every 36 hours, so that in the common form of acute *noncorrosive* gastritis, the problem is usually relatively brief —unless the precipitating cause is still present to continue doing what it did originally: produce inflammation and erosion and sometimes small hemorrhages in the mucous lining.

If you eliminate the cause, symptoms usually disappear within 48 hours. So remove the offending material, whatever it may be—aspirin, alcohol, a specific food or set of foods.

Special diet is not needed. Often, nausea and vomiting may prevent eating anyway. If the nausea and vomiting are severe, your physician can prescribe a drug such as prochlorperazine. If they are not too severe, an over-the-counter preparation such as Emetrol may help. Antacids may help to relieve pain. Usually, a nonabsorbable antacid in liquid form—such as Maalox, Gelusil, or Mylanta—is best.

Gastroenteritis, Acute

An acute inflammation of the lining of the stomach and intestine, acute gastroenteritis can be caused by a virus ("intestinal grippe," "intestinal flu"), overindulgence in alcohol, food allergy, food poisoning, various drugs (such as salicylates or aspirinlike compounds, quinacrine, colchicine), heavy metals (arsenic, lead, mercury, cadmium), and infectious diseases.

The inflammation develops suddenly. The nature and severity of symptoms depend on the irritant, how much of the gastrointestinal tract is affected, and the general health and resistance of the individual.

Commonly, however, there is some degree of malaise, appetite loss, nausea, vomiting, cramps, gut rumbling, and diarrhea. In severe cases, prostration may occur and blood and mucus may appear in stools. If the gastroenteritis is infectious in origin, fever often develops.

WHAT TO DO: Often, symptoms subside within 48 hours. During that time, bed rest is advisable. Eating and drinking are well avoided until nausea and vomiting subside. Then, in order to replace the fluid and salt the body has lost, light fluids such as tea and strained broth, bouillon with added salt, and cereal can be taken. When these are tolerated, other foods such as eggs, gelatin, and simple puddings may be added.

If vomiting persists, an antiemetic agent such as Emetrol, available without prescription, may help. To prevent dangerous dehydration from the vomiting, fluids are needed. If water can't be taken, a carbonated beverage may go down and stay down; otherwise cracked ice may be sucked. If vomiting continues, medical help to control it is needed and, if necessary, fluids may have to be given by vein. If diarrhea is persistent, an agent such as Kaopectate or paregoric can be used.

Food Infection Gastroenteritis

This is the result of eating food contaminated by such bacteria as salmonellae, streptococci, or *E. coli.*

Symptoms develop from 6 to 48 hours after eating. They include headache, chills, fever, muscle aches, nausea, vomiting, cramps, diarrhea, and prostration. In severe cases, stools and vomitus may contain blood.

Usually the illness is over in 24 to 48 hours, and sometimes it can be mild enough so the patient goes about usual activities during its course.

WHAT TO DO: Treatment is the same as just discussed for acute gastroenteritis. In severe cases, your physician may prescribe an antibiotic. Try to recall a food you have eaten in the past two days that might have caused the infection. It could be a raw or inadequately cooked food or a cold dish made with mayonnaise and left out at warm temperature. If you suspect a culprit, you can warn others who ate the same food, and the information could help your physician to consider the possible bacteria and establish the best treatment for yourself and others.

Staphylococcus Toxin Gastroenteritis

This sometimes violent upset, one of the most common forms of food poisoning, is caused by a toxic material produced by staphylococcal bacteria growing in such foods as milk, cream-filled pastries, custards, and processed meat and fish. Improperly supervised food handlers are largely responsible.

Symptoms—nausea, vomiting, cramps, diarrhea, and sometimes headache and fever—usually develop within two to four hours after the contaminated food is eaten.

The attack is brief, often lasting only three to six hours, and recovery is complete. Treatment, if needed, is the same as for acute gastroenteritis.

Food Poisoning Requiring Immediate Medical Help

BOTULISM: Almost always caused by improperly canned (or otherwise preserved) foods in which a bacillus produces a toxin, botulism causes symptoms anywhere from four hours to eight days after the food is eaten. They begin with fatigue and lassitude, shortly followed by visual disturbances and then by muscle weakening and swallowing difficulty. Vomiting and diarrhea occur in about one third of the cases.

The botulism death rate is high, 65 percent, with most deaths occurring between the second and ninth days, from breathing paralysis or pneumonia. Hospitalization is essential. Botulism antiserum is administered. Saliva must be sucked out of the mouth when the patient cannot swallow. Intravenous feeding may be needed for several days. A respirator is used if there is a threat to breathing.

NONBACTERIAL FOOD POISONING: Some species of *mushrooms* contain a poison which, within minutes to two hours, produces cramps, diarrhea, confusion, sweating, collapse, and sometimes convulsions. The poison of some other species causes liver damage, jaundice, low blood pressure, racing pulse, and subnormal temperature. Mushroom poisoning can be fatal in as many as 50 percent of cases.

Immature and sprouting potatoes may contain a toxic compound, *solanine*, that within a few hours of ingestion produces nausea, vomiting, cramps, diarrhea, throat constriction, pupil dilation, and prostration. Virtually all victims recover.

Some *clams and mussels*, especially on the Pacific coast, may, from June to October, ingest an organism that produces a toxin not destroyed by cooking. Symptoms, within 5 to 30 minutes, include nausea, vomiting, cramps, muscle weakness, and paralysis. Sometimes death may occur because of breathing failure.

Ergot poisoning—from eating rye or other grain contaminated with a fungus—may produce such symptoms as chest pain, heartbeat disturbances, weakness, headache, itching, painful cramps in the extremities, gangrene of toes or fingers, and epilepticlike convulsions.

Fava bean poisoning (favism), which may occur in those sensitive to the bean, produces dizziness, vomiting, diarrhea, prostration, and anemia.

Medical treatment for nonbacterial food poisoning may include bed rest, washing out the stomach, drugs for pain, injection of fluids to combat dehydration. Other drugs—to relieve blood vessel spasm or convulsions when present—may be used.

Giardiasis (See WORM-INDUCED DISEASES)

Glands, Swollen

Lymph nodes, commonly referred to as *lymph glands*, are strategically located throughout the body and are part of the body's defense system.

When infectious organisms invade the body, white cells in

the blood multiply, move to the infected area, attack and devour the organisms. The infected area becomes a mass of living and dead organisms and white cells, which form the pus that develops in infected tissue. The debris is moved to the lymph nodes where it is filtered and gradually destroyed. That is why swollen lymph nodes are indicators of infection.

Often, you can identify the location of the infection that is producing the swelling. Sore throats and ear infections are often accompanied by swelling of nodes in the neck; infec-

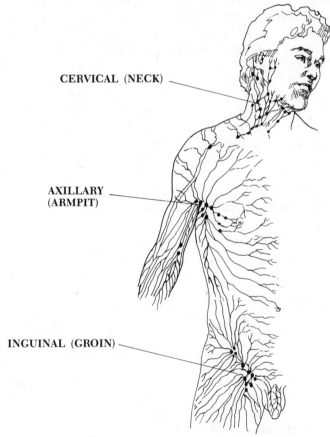

CERVICAL (NECK)

AXILLARY
(ARMPIT)

INGUINAL (GROIN)

Fig. 21. Lymph glands (nodes).

tions in the genital area or legs, by swelling of nodes in the groin.

WHAT TO DO: When obvious infection is present, there will be other symptoms such as fever, pain, possibly redness, depending upon the site. The node swellings themselves should be of no concern except as a warning of infection elsewhere. The specific infection needs treatment. (see CUTS; EARACHE; THROAT, SORE.)

Sometimes, nodes are swollen when only a very minor, not obvious infection is present.

When nodes swell without apparent reason and there are no other symptoms, you can check with your physician then or delay checking with him for a week or two while watching the swellings carefully. If they persist, the physician can look for hidden infections or other possible causes, usually not grave.

It should be noted, however, that the nodes also serve to help stop cancer fr u spreading by filtering out malignant cells. In the absence of infection, large nodes that are not tender may have to be removed in a minor surgical procedure to determine the cause of swelling.

Gonorrhea (See VENEREAL DISEASES)

Gout

If you wake up some night with a painful toe, it could be your first attack of gout. It is more likely to be gout if you're male, if the pain has a certain nature I will describe, and if you note some other signs to be discussed here.

A first acute attack of gout usually appears without warning. Night is the favorite time but it can occur at other times. The big toe is the favorite site but sometimes the wrist, ankle or thumb joint may be affected. Gout can attack women but 95 percent of victims are men.

Ordinary arthritis produces pain that is deep and aching,

but with gout the pain is sharp, often described as crushing, throbbing, excruciating. It becomes progressively more severe. Even the weight of the lightest clothes or bedcovering cannot be tolerated.

The toe or other affected joint becomes swollen, shiny, warm, red or purplish in color. And there may be fever, chills, malaise.

A gout attack may be triggered by minor injury (such as from ill-fitting shoes), food or alcohol overindulgence, fatigue, infection, treatment with some drugs (penicillin, insulin, diuretics or "water pills"). Excessive loss of body water (dehydration) as a result of a hard game of tennis or other vigorous activity may contribute.

What's involved is an excess of uric acid in body fluids. When uric acid is in excess, it can form crystals of sodium urate which are deposited in and around joints and tendons.

WHAT TO DO: Without treatment, a first attack of gout may last several agonizing days.

If you suspect you are having a gout attack, get in touch with your physician as quickly as possible. He can prescribe an antiinflammatory drug.

Colchicine is the drug of choice, especially for a first attack. Made from the autumn crocus, colchicine has been known for more than a thousand years.

It's a remarkable drug for gout—first, because of the dramatic response it produces, making pain subside after 12 hours and disappear completely within 36 to 48 hours. It has another value: because it is of little or no use for anything but gout, response to it helps to confirm the diagnosis of gout.

The dose of colchicine is about 0.6 milligram by mouth every hour until relief begins or vomiting or diarrhea occurs. A severe episode may require from 4 to 7 milligrams.

Also effective are two other antiinflammatory agents—phenylbutazone and indomethacin—either of which your physician may prescribe and either of which is especially valuable for people who cannot tolerate colchicine.

Going Further: Once an acute attack is over, preventive measures are needed. Without them, repeated attacks are likely to occur. As chronic gout develops, urates can be deposited in other parts of the body such as the earlobes and in various joints and tendons, producing hard, painless tumors called *tophi*. If crystals should be deposited in the kidneys, kidney damage can follow. In addition, excess uric acid in the urine can produce kidney stones.

Prophylactic measures can markedly reduce or even eliminate acute attacks and prevent the development of chronic gout.

One or more of several drugs may be used. Colchicine in small daily doses, much lower than for an acute attack, is valuable. There are *uricosuric drugs* which help by increasing the excretion of uric acid; they include probenecid and sulfinpyrazone. Their proper daily dosage can be determined by blood tests which indicate when uric acid is down to a desirable level.

Another valuable drug is allopurinol, which works to block the production of uric acid.

Once gout victims had to live with diet restrictions, banning foods that produce large amounts of uric acid. Now drugs are so effective that restrictions are often not considered necessary.

Although drugs provide relief, there may, in some cases, as with all medications, be side effects. It is usually said that once on a drug for gout, attacks will recur when the drug is stopped. A personal experience, shared by some other physicians, albeit not a scientific evaluation, warrants noting. By keeping up an adequate intake of fluids and increasing fluid intake at the first sign of joint discomfort, I have been able to forestall symptoms, eliminating the need for drugs.

Hangover

The only respite from hangover is usually found in the often-repeated words, "Never again!" Despite many efforts to discover some panacea, or sure cure, none exists.

But there are some possibly helpful suggestions based on recent neurological studies of the hangover phenomenon.

WHAT TO DO: The throbbing headache of hangover results from dilation of blood vessels in the head induced by alcohol. Migraine preparations containing caffeine and ergotamine, or the caffeine in black coffee, may help to relieve the headache because of a constricting effect on blood vessels.

Alcohol tends to dehydrate. But if you try to drink water to quench thirst and replace body fluids, nausea may be aggravated. Instead, several cups of salted beef broth taken at intervals will replace both fluid and lost minerals and may help ease nausea.

Alcohol is metabolized and used up by the body at a constant rate. But fructose—a natural sugar occurring in ripe fruits, honey, vegetables, and extracts such as tomato juice—may be useful in accelerating the metabolism of alcohol and thus possibly speeding the departure of the hangover.

Not least of all, being erect helps to reduce blood vessel dilation; lying in bed does not.

Hay Fever (See ALLERGIES)

Headaches

It would be difficult to conceive of a more unlikely cause of puzzling headaches than bedcovers—more accurately, sleeping with bedcovers over the head. Yet such headaches, aptly named "turtle" headaches, have been reported in a series of patients—and until identified for what they are they can be quite mysterious, awakening victims from sleep during the night or striking upon arising in the morning, generalized, the whole head hurting. The cure is simple enough: Give up the covers-over-the-head habit that apparently causes headache by depriving the brain of adequate oxygen.

Headaches, of course, can accompany many diseases along with other symptoms, such as fever, muscle aches and pains in flu.

But headache without any other associated symptoms is most commonly of the tension or muscle contraction type in which, usually as the result of emotional or other stress but sometimes because of strained posture (as in driving in a rainstorm, for example), neck, and scalp, and even jaw muscles may go into spasm. For such headaches, aspirin is often helpful, especially if coupled with other measures such as massage or heat applied to the back of the neck and resting with eyes closed and the head supported.

Recently, for some sufferers with often-repeated tension headaches, biofeedback has been found useful. If you belong in this category, you may want to try feedback, which essentially is a method of relaxation now being offered in many hospital headache clinics. Typically, electrodes are placed on the forehead (a totally painless procedure) to record muscle tension. With tension level high, the biofeedback equipment may emit rapid beeps. As tension is reduced, the beeps come more slowly. And as you learn—in some fashion difficult to explain—to make the beeps slow down, with the aid of the biofeedback equipment, you note what you are doing to achieve the feat and then may be able to reproduce it without the equipment, as a means of stopping a headache before it has time to really get started.

MIGRAINE: Many of what are called migraine headaches are really severe tension headaches and would better be treated that way. True migraine headaches often are preceded by visual disturbances such as "seeing stars" and accompanied by nausea. They affect one side of the head, although the side may vary from one attack to another. Migraine headaches involve constriction and relaxation of blood vessels in the head. Drugs that affect blood vessels, such as Cafergot, may help migraine but not tension headaches.

If you're a migraine victim, you may not have been getting adequate relief from medications such as Cafergot. The problem may lie with taking medication when nausea is already present; when nausea is present, the stomach often absorbs medication poorly. One maneuver you may find helpful in determining whether a migraine or another kind of headache is coming is to sit down and place your head between your knees. If the head throbs, a migraine episode is very probably on its way, and medication for it should be taken immediately.

Is diet involved in migraine? Recent research does suggest that certain foods can, in the migraine-prone, have an effect on blood vessels that may trigger attacks. They include red wines and champagne, aged or strong cheese (particularly cheddar), pickled herring, chicken livers, pods of broad beans, and canned figs. Their avoidance may be helpful.

For some people, cured meats, including frankfurters, bacon, ham, and salami, may have adverse effects, and a trial of avoiding them may be worthwhile. Monosodium glutamate, a salt used to enhance the flavor of foods, may in large amounts trigger migraine, and excesses should be avoided.

Recently, too, biofeedback has been used with reported success to reduce the frequency and intensity of migraine headaches. There has also been some success for people unresponsive to usual migraine medications with propranolol, a drug often used for heart patients, and, in other cases, with amitriptyline, an antidepressant drug often used for mental depression.

OTHER HEADACHES: Nitrites are chemical compounds that may be used as preservatives in cured meats, and at least one recent study indicates that in some people sensitive to nitrites they may be responsible for otherwise mysterious headaches —moderately severe, nonthrobbing, usually lasting several hours and sometimes accompanied by facial flushing. If you happen to be sensitive to nitrites, such headaches may occur within half an hour after eating such cured meat products as frankfurters, bacon, salami, and ham, which contain the compounds.

Caffeinism—excessive intake of caffeine in the form of coffee, tea, cola drinks, and even medications that contain caffeine—has been linked with some cases of what appear to be severe, recurrent tension headaches. If you're a frequent headache sufferer and also a heavy partaker of caffeine, you may want to try minimizing your caffeine intake to see if that helps.

Persistent headaches that do not respond to any of the measures you can try at home should have medical attention—

preferably the kind of expert attention you may get from a physician or clinic specializing in headache diagnosis and treatment. Chances are, if you inquire, you can find such a physician or clinic not too far from you.

Head Injuries

No injury to the head, however seemingly slight or trivial, should be ignored.

It may or may not be serious.

If you observe certain guidelines, you can avoid needless anxiety, on the one hand, and neglect of something serious, on the other.

Typically, in a *minor* head injury, there may be a quickly developing bump, some initial stunning, but no loss of consciousness. Especially in a child, there may even be an episode of vomiting or two in the first few hours, which then stops. Not long afterward, all is well except perhaps the swollen bump, which will disappear in due course.

WHAT TO DO FOR MINOR INJURY: Apply ice as soon as possible to minimize the size of the swelling. If there is a bleeding scalp wound—and scalp wounds tend to bleed profusely—raise the victim's head and shoulders to control the bleeding. Apply a sterile dressing snugly on the wound, and when bleeding is under control, bandage the dressing to hold it in place.

WHAT TO DO FOR MORE SEVERE INJURY: In a more *severe* injury, there may be immediate or delayed indications.

Get medical help without delay if a clear or blood-tinged fluid drains from the nose and ear; it may indicate a skull fracture. Get medical help, too, in case of unconsciousness.

Until medical help is available, keep the victim lying down. Lying quietly helps to lessen the possibility or extent of hemorrhage within the skull.

If the victim is unconscious or having difficulty breathing, turn his head gently to the side to allow blood or mucus to drain from the corner of the mouth.

A valuable trick if you are alone with a person who has a scalp laceration: Use the victim's hair as a suture (stitch).

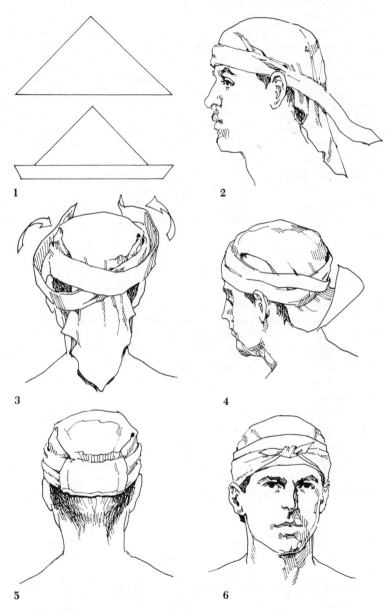

Fig. 22. Applying a dressing for head injury.

Take a few hairs on each side of the cut and tie them to each other, so the edges of the wound are pulled together, closing it and controlling the bleeding. Tie three knots in each set of hair strands. Repeat with other strands until the wound is closed. The knots may tend to pull apart if the hair is oily; if you have collodion available, touch some to the knots and hold until the collodion sticks. Then apply a sterile dressing.

Note: Even in the absence of potentially serious indications such as fluid draining from the nose and ear or unconsciousness, anyone who has had more than a very mild head injury should restrict activity for 24 hours and not be left alone.

And a watch should be kept for any of the following signs, which may indicate possible brain damage:

• Variable consciousness: Periods of drowsiness interspersed with alertness can indicate increasing pressure on the brain.

• Increasing lethargy, excessive sleepiness, difficulty of arousal require a call for a physician.

• The pupils of the eyes—the small black circles inside the colored rings in the center of the eyes—should be the same size in both eyes and should contract in size when a light is shined into the eyes. If they are unequal in size and fail to contract when exposed to light, there may be increased brain pressure and urgent need for medical help.

• Irrational or unusual behavior, including unusual restlessness, may be a warning.

• Severe, recurrent, and often forceful vomiting calls for medical help.

• Irregular, slow, and deep breathing may indicate increased brain pressure and need for medical attention.

• Arm or leg muscle weakness, drooping of an eye or one side of the mouth, or tingling, numbness or paralysis in one arm or leg may indicate brain damage and need for medical help.

• A change of vision, particularly blurring or double vision, if it persists, calls for medical attention.

• Persistent or severe headache may mean serious injury— but note that after any head injury headache is not unusual. An ordinary headache, however, usually tends to gradually decrease rather than intensify. Apply an ice pack or cold wet towel and use aspirin if needed but avoid anything stronger —and if these measures do nothing for the headache, medical help is probably needed.

Note: Sometimes, days or weeks after a head injury and an apparently good recovery, there may be late changes indicating trouble. Some confusion, a change in personality (often slight), and increasing somnolence may indicate a slowly increasing blood clot within the skull (subdural hematoma) which is compressing the brain and requires medical attention.

REMEMBER:

1. Control scalp bleeding; it can be profuse.
2. Careful observation is necessary to recognize complications early.
3. Clear or blood-tinged fluid from nose or ear may indicate a skull fracture.

Heart Attack

A prime symptom of a heart attack is chest pain. It may range from a slight feeling of pressure to a sensation of having the chest crushed in a vise.

Someone who has been having attacks of angina (the chest pain associated with coronary heart disease) may think at first that he is having another angina episode. But, with a heart attack, stopping activity does not help, as it does with angina. Typically, the chest pain of a heart attack persists and will not subside until a narcotic such as morphine is administered.

With the pain, almost always there is a feeling of tremendous anxiety, a sense of foreboding that death is near. The face often turns ashen gray and a cold sweat develops. Sometimes, retching, belching and vomiting occur—one reason why a heart attack may sometimes be confused with a stomach upset. Shortness of breath is common, and palpitations may occur.

WHAT TO DO: Because the first hours and sometimes even minutes can be critical in dealing with a heart attack, if you have the slightest suspicion you may be having one, get yourself taken to the nearest hospital emergency room or have someone summon a rescue squad. Immediately on arrival at a hospital, tell personnel you may be having a heart attack and insist on being taken to a coronary care unit.

If you are not the victim but are trying to help someone who is, or may be, having a heart attack, act calmly but expeditiously. Get help as quickly as possible; call an ambulance or rescue squad. When a telephone call is impossible, take the victim to the nearest hospital emergency room.

Although there is little you can do to help the victim directly unless you have special training, you can help by making certain there are no obstructions in the mouth or at the throat that might interfere with breathing.

If you are skilled in cardiopulmonary resuscitation (CPR), you should use your training if it becomes necessary to do so because of breathing or heart stoppage. CPR should not be entered into lightly, however, as serious injuries have been reported in some cases when it has been used, even in people not suffering heart attacks.

A cardinal point to remember—and a reassuring one: Most heart attacks do not kill immediately, do not involve massive destruction of heart tissue. A major risk is that even with a relatively minor heart attack, a disturbance of heart rhythm may develop within minutes or hours. If detected and treated in time, the disturbance can be corrected before it has a chance to become a potentially lethal disturbance. This may require drug treatment or use of an electrical current to restore normal rhythm—and monitoring for and correcting abnormal heart rhythms are routine in coronary care units, which is why heart attack victims have the best chance when they reach and remain in such units.

Heartbeat Irregularities

Palpitation

This is a word that covers a lot of territory. It means a heartbeat that is unusually rapid, strong or irregular enough to make you aware of it.

There are, of course, palpitations that result from heart disorders. In most cases, however, palpitations arise because of excitement or nervousness, extreme exertion, fatigue, medications, or an excess of caffeine.

Following, more precisely defined, are the more common heartbeat irregularities.

Extra Heartbeat

Also known as *extrasystole, premature beat,* and *skipped beat,* this can involve what may seem to be an alarming flutter or jump in the chest, a feeling of a skipped beat or extra beat but no pain.

It can be produced by fatigue, tension, excessive intake of tea or coffee, chocolate, smoking, or an unusual medication. It is usually not serious and has no damaging effect on the heart if there is no heart disease. Often, in a healthy heart, exercise may eliminate the extra beat.

WHAT TO DO: Especially if the extra beats persist and/or you have other reasons to suspect you may have a heart problem, see a physician. Persistent extra beats can be eliminated with medication.

Rapid Heartbeat

A rapid heartbeat—over 100 times a minute—is often caused simply by exertion or excitement. It sometimes may occur with menstruation, pregnancy, or menopause.

Many drugs can produce rapid beating—among them, adrenaline, amphetamines, and belladonna—and overindulgence in coffee, tea or other caffeine-containing beverages, as well as alcohol, can speed up the heart.

Rapid heartbeat also can be associated with physical problems—anemia, infectious disease, hyperthroidism (excessive thyroid gland activity), Addison's disease, heart disorder, and low blood sugar.

WHAT TO DO: If you experience persistent or repeated episodes of rapid beating which is not linked to exertion or excitement or to drugs and overindulgences (and not relieved when you avoid these), you should have a physician check for an organic problem that requires treatment.

Paroxysmal Tachycardia

This is a kind of rapid heartbeat, as high as 180 or even higher, which can appear suddenly, often without known cause. It may persist for hours or even days, stop just as suddenly as it appeared, and then reappear at another time. When the beat is extremely rapid, there may be such symptoms as pallor, nausea, weakness, fainting, and sometimes even shock.

WHAT TO DO: Often, an attack of paroxysmal tachycardia can be stopped by any of several maneuvers.

One is to lie down with feet higher than head. Another is to bend forward from the waist as far as you can. Still another is to try closing the larynx, or voice box, and make an effort to breathe out against it. Applying pressure (not excessive) on both eyeballs sometimes helps. So does induced vomiting.

If these fail, a physician can use drugs to stop the attack.

Slow Heartbeat

Actually, a slow heartbeat—of about 50 beats or even a little less per minute—is an indication of top form in an athlete or someone who maintains excellent physical fitness.

But there are some heart disorders, some infectious diseases, and sometimes diabetes which may lead to slow beat, and if the beat becomes very slow it may cause fainting.

WHAT TO DO: If you suddenly begin to experience a slow beat—one not associated with good physical fitness achieved after extensive training—you should have a physician check for and treat the cause.

Atrial Fibrillation

This is a rapid, continuous but irregular, fluttering heartbeat which can produce pallor, weakness, and a strange feeling in the chest.

Rarely, atrial fibrillation can appear in a healthy person.

Usually, it is associated with a heart problem or with excessive thyroid gland function.

WHAT TO DO: See a physician. The fibrillation and the underlying problem may be treated with various drugs. And the outlook is usually good.

Ventricular Fibrillation

This is a totally disorganized kind of beating—in fact, not so much a beating of the heart as a useless twitching and fluttering, rapid, weak, the heart working but unable to pump blood.

This is a grave emergency. Ventricular fibrillation can be brought on by a heart attack or an overdose of heart drugs.

Symptoms include total collapse, absence of pulse, pallor.

Most hospitals—and now many ambulances and rescue teams—have an electrical device, a *defibrillator*, that can shock the heart back to normal rhythm through electrodes placed on the chest.

Until help arrives, there is no choice but to try—and work earnestly at—CPR (cardiopulmonary resuscitation). (See p. 52.) Begin CPR immediately and continue until help arrives.

Heartburn

A very common problem, heartburn affects about half the population occasionally, while 20 percent suffer from it chronically.

It's a burning sensation deep in the chest, similar to what you might expect if you were to swallow a hot coal. Along with the burning, there is an oppressive tightening sensation. The discomfort can extend from the lower end of the breastbone up to the throat, following the course of the esophagus or gullet.

Gas is often present, and commonly there are efforts, often successful, to belch. But if TV commercials make it seem that gas is the primary cause of heartburn, it is not.

Heartburn involves reflux, or abnormal return, of material, including acid, from the stomach into the esophagus. Out of place in the esophagus, which does not have the stomach's protection against it, the acid produces a painful reaction.

It used to be believed that reflux was caused by hiatus hernia (see HERNIA, HIATUS). But not all people with hiatus hernia have heartburn, and some with severe heartburn have no hiatus hernia.

The problem lies in an area about an inch long at the lower end of the esophagus where it joins the stomach. The area— called the *lower esophageal sphincter (LES)*—acts like a valve, opening to allow food to pass down into the stomach, then closing behind.

Heartburn occurs when LES pressure is below normal, so the sphincter does not close tightly enough and there is less of a barrier against reflux.

Even in the face of some reduction of LES pressure, heartburn is not a constant problem. Certain factors promote it.

One is a large meal. Overfilling the stomach may create pressures within the stomach sufficient to overcome the weakened LES ability to stay closed.

Lying down within an hour or two after a meal, when the stomach still may be full, also can encourage heartburn, since it removes the downward pull of gravity on stomach contents, and they may then slip through the LES more readily.

Also, it is natural for the abdomen to distend after a meal; this, in fact, reduces pressures within the abdomen and, in doing so, reduces the likelihood of reflux. But a tight belt or tight clothing can interfere with normal distention and trigger heartburn. Obesity, too, tends to increase pressures within the abdomen, and weight loss is often helpful for people frequently bothered with heartburn.

Some foods may cause heartburn for some people, and there may be individual idiosyncrasies about the specific foods. But recent studies in which measurements have actually been made of LES pressure indicate that alcohol, chocolate, and fat may often be involved, since they do reduce sphincter pressure. Smoking does the same.

WHAT TO DO: If you experience heartburn frequently, attention to one or more of the preceding factors may help to solve your problem. If not, should you resort to antacids?

Antacids can help. They neutralize acid. Additionally, there is some evidence now that they may increase LES pressure. Liquid antacids are more effective than tablets, even if not as convenient.

Some people resort to bicarbonate of soda in the form of baking soda. And many commonly sold tablet preparations are primarily composed of sodium bicarbonate. Bicarbonate will neutralize acid in the stomach temporarily and, by creating carbon dioxide gas, will provide enough gas to permit belching. The so-called relief from belching would not be necessary if the bicarbonate were not taken in the first place. Chronic resort to bicarbonate may cause increased acid formation in the stomach. The sodium, too, may not be advisable for people with high blood pressure or a heart problem. Some tablets also contain aspirin, not a drug to be taken needlessly.

A promising development for people who suffer chronically from severe heartburn is a drug, bethanechol, which has been found to have a marked LES-pressure-increasing effect and often provides relief. Your physician can prescribe it.

Heat Collapse (See HEAT PROSTRATION)

Heat Cramp

Appearing abruptly and excruciatingly painful, heat cramps most often affect the arms and legs but sometimes may involve the abdominal muscles. Wherever they occur, they are muscle cramps that occur in paroxysms with relative comfort in between.

The cramps are caused by failure to replace salt lost during profuse perspiration accompanying heavy exertion at air temperatures usually greater than 100°F or 38° Celsius. They have also occurred in springtime in novice skiers who sweat profusely because they are dressed too warmly with insulated garments. In a dry desert climate, you may not feel wet but may lose even more perspiration than when you are aware of the loss.

WHAT TO DO: To help relieve the spasm, massage the cramped muscles gently. If that fails to help, try exerting firm pressure with your hand. Do *NOT* use hot packs.

At the same time, start sipping salt water—about half a glass containing half a teaspoonful of salt—every 15 minutes and continue for an hour.

Usually these measures work. In extreme cases, an emergency room physician can administer an intravenous infusion of a salt solution (isotonic saline).

PREVENTION: If you know you are going to be doing heavy work or exercise under high temperature conditions, you can prevent cramps by taking 1 or 2 grams of salt with water four times a day.

Heat Prostration (Heat Exhaustion)

Also called *heat collapse*, this condition results from failure to adjust to prolonged exposure to high heat.

Often before the attack, there are warning symptoms: weakness, dizziness, nausea, headache, blurring or dimming of vision, mild muscle cramps.

With the attack, the skin becomes damp, cold, and ashen, and there may be profuse sweating. Listlessness and apprehension are common, and sometimes there may be a semicomatose or unconscious state.

WHAT TO DO: Lie down—if possible in a cool place. Loosen clothing. Sip water, preferably with salt in it, half a teaspoonful to half a glass of water. In the absence of a cool place, apply cool wet cloths.

If profound collapse has occurred, medical attention is needed. In a hospital emergency room, a slow intravenous infusion of salt solution (isotonic salt solution) can be administered; and if needed, oxygen, heart stimulants, and other medication can be given.

Usually heat prostration is transient and the outlook excellent. A danger in severe prostration is failure of blood circulation, but this can be corrected by emergency room measures.

PREVENTION: As much as possible, avoid heavy exertion and profuse sweating under conditions of high heat, especially if you are not used to the heat. Note, too, that the likelihood of prostration is increased by drinking alcohol or after vomiting or diarrhea, either of which can dehydrate the body.

Drink plenty of water or other fluids before and during exposure. Usually, it is best to wear loose and light clothing. Increase your salt intake, too, by taking 1 or 2 grams of salt with water four times a day.

Heat Rash (See MILIARIA)

Heatstroke (Sunstroke)

This is a severe disturbance of the body's heat-regulating system caused by prolonged exposure to heat or sunshine, sometimes combined with strenuous exertion. It can occur in anyone but has a higher incidence in older people and those with heart, lung, or other chronic disease. It is more common on the second day of a heat wave.

Symptoms may follow warning indications such as weakness, headache, dizziness, appetite loss, nausea, and distress over the heart and stomach area. Sometimes, several hours before the attack, sweating may diminish or stop entirely. But the symptoms in some cases may appear abruptly without such warnings.

The skin is hot, flushed, dry; fever is obvious. The temperature rises quickly to 105° or 106°F or higher. Muscle cramps or twitching may occur. The pulse rate may go to 160 or higher.

WHAT TO DO: *Heatstroke is a grave threat to life.* Medical attention as quickly as possible is needed.

Until such attention is available, you can do these things:

Bring temperature down. Give aspirin, 10 grains, by mouth or rectal suppository. Undress the victim. Sponge with cool water or rubbing alcohol or apply cold packs.

If body temperature is above 106°F, cover the victim with a blanket soaked in cold water or give a cold tub bath, massaging vigorously until temperature falls.

But note carefully: As you work to bring down body temperature, check temperature rectally every 10 minutes and *BRING DOWN ONLY TO 101°, NOT LOWER.* The reason is that the temperature may continue to fall to a dangerous level. At 101°, stop cold applications of any kind, have the victim stay in bed, in a cool, well-ventilated room (even exposed to an electric fan). *And continue massage,* because it helps to counter the constriction of blood vessels produced by the cold and helps to get cooler blood flowing to the brain.

If temperature rises again, repeat cooling procedure.

To supplement such vital immediate treatment, a physician can use other measures as needed: administration of fluids with bicarbonate and other medication, by vein.

Heel Pain

Common causes of painful heel include bursitis due to ill-fitting shoes, and bruising or inflammation of ligaments from undue strain. Often flatfoot is a contributing factor and may need correction with the aid of sponge rubber, metal, or plastic arch supports.

An increase in shoe heel height may be used temporarily to relieve strain on the Achilles tendon at the back of the heel, which connects calf muscles to the heel bone.

To relieve pressure on a painful spot under the heel, a felt or sponge rubber ring pad can be used. Warm soaks and massage are often helpful.

Jumping from a height of a few feet and landing flatfooted can cause a fracture of the heel bones, requiring orthopedic treatment.

Chronic heel pain may sometimes be due to a bone spur that must be removed by surgery.

Hemorrhoids (Piles)

Hemorrhoids, or piles, are expanded veins, varicose-type, under the mucous membrane lining of the anal and rectal area. When they occur in the wall of the rectum above the sphincter muscle, they are classified as *internal;* those below, in the anal canal, are called *external.* Often, both internal and external hemorrhoids may be present.

External hemorrhoids may be soft and painless, although they may cause a sense of fullness at the anus. Sometimes, under acute local stress—such as straining at stool to overcome constipation or, alternatively, following diarrhea—the veins may suddenly enlarge, become filled with blood clots and inflamed, and may break down and bleed. The condition is extremely painful, more so during bowel movements, usually lasts for about five days until the clots begin to be absorbed and the mass disappears. After such an attack, there may be no symptoms or there may be severe itching.

Internal hemorrhoids may bleed as the result of minor injuries, and bleeding is usually the main symptom. But if the hemorrhoids are large, there may be a feeling of incomplete evacuation of the rectum.

Many factors can contribute to the development and exacerbation of hemorrhoids.

The veins may become distended in people who habitually have to stand or sit for long periods—hemorrhoids are a common problem in bus, taxi, and truck drivers, for example.

Hemorrhoids can be a problem during pregnancy when the enlarging uterus may press on blood vessels in the abdomen and cause some reduction of normal blood flow back to the heart from veins in the rectal area, which then become distended. Hemorrhoids that appear during pregnancy, fortunately, usually disappear after delivery.

During bowel movement, all parts of the anorectal area, including the veins, are stretched, but after passage of the stool, they return to a normal relaxed state. If, however, the veins are weak, as may be the case in some people, they tend to remain stretched.

A major factor in hemorrhoid development and exacerbation is increased pressure within the vein system. This may be produced sometimes by obesity, coughing, or sneezing. But a major source is straining at stool because of constipation. People who are chronically constipated and are always straining at stool build considerable pressure and push out the veins.

Rough and irritating toilet paper may make hemorrhoids worse.

WHAT TO DO: If you are suffering from a painful hemorrhoid attack, one of the best things you can do is to take a *sitz bath*—which simply means sitting in a warm tub. If the hemorrhoids itch, adding a cupful of cornstarch to a tub of water may help. Aspirin also may help to relieve the pain and inflammation.

If at this point you are passing large, hard stools, the temporary use of mineral oil to soften them may help. Take two to four tablespoons of mineral oil two to three times a day—but only to overcome an acute attack. Constant use of mineral oil can diminish the body's ability to absorb some important vitamins. Also helpful for the same purpose of stool softening: drink a lot of fluids.

If constipation is your problem—right now during an attack and at other times as well, making it an important or even the only factor in the hemorrhoid condition—you may do well to add fiber to your diet. The lack of it is a major cause of constipation (see CONSTIPATION).

Do you need any of the commercial suppositories or ointments? Usually not, if you follow the foregoing suggestions. If these suggestions prove inadequate or for any reason you are unable to follow them, the commercial preparations may help a little, giving slight, temporary relief of itching, pain, and inflammation.

When external hemorrhoids become clotted, the pain usually stops within three to five days, and the mass is gone within three to four weeks. If you find the pain intolerable, the clots can be quickly removed by a physician, using a local anesthetic to make a small incision, which gives immediate relief.

SURGERY: If the itching or pain of hemorrhoids is long-lasting and severe, or if bleeding is severe and persistent to the point of leading to anemia, you may consider surgery.

But when examination such as barium enema x-ray and looking into the rectum and colon have established that there is no tumor present and causing the bleeding, avoid a rush to surgery. Operation is not necessary is most persons with hemorrhoids. Control of the constipation or diarrhea, as previously mentioned, will in most cases make surgery unnecessary.

Hemorrhoidectomy, as the standard operation for hemorrhoids is called, involves tying off the hemorrhoids close to their origin, carefully dissecting them out, and removing them. It is relatively simple, not considered major surgery, takes on the average about half an hour or less, and can be performed under general, spinal, or caudal anesthesia.

For as long as five days afterward, there may be considerable pain. For relief, local anesthetics may be applied and daily sitz baths used.

Usually, the patient is out of bed the day after the operation, home in 4 days, and the rectal area becomes completely painless in 10 to 14 days. Once successfully removed, hemorrhoids cannot recur, and the permanent cure rate is greater than 90 percent. Sometimes, however, other veins may enlarge if the causative factors are not remedied.

AN ALTERNATIVE PROCEDURE: Although not all hemorrhoids, particularly complicated ones, are suitable for it, a nonsurgical procedure called *rubber-band ligation* is being used increasingly by many surgeons.

It involves placing a special latex band over the neck of a hemorrhoid. The band ties off the hemorrhoid, which then gets no blood, dries up, and usually falls off in 1 to 14 days. No general anesthesia is needed; the procedure is essentially painless and can be performed in a doctor's office. Usually, only one ligation is done in the office on each occasion, since it may be difficult to do a second with the first obstructing the view. Subsequent ligations may be done at two-week intervals or sooner.

Although pain after ligation is not common, there usually is some discomfort—a sensation of rectal fullness and urge to defecate. When the hemorrhoid drops off, there may be some brief blood spotting; rarely is there serious bleeding. Itching may be aggravated for a time when the hemorrhoid drops off.

Hepatitis, Acute Viral

A common acute infectious disease of the liver, acute viral hepatitis (*hepar-*, liver; *-itis*, inflammation or infection) is caused by a virus that enters via the mouth, spread by person-to-person contact and by fecally contaminated food and water.

The disease, also known as *hepatitis A*, often can be so mild that there is no awareness of its presence, although it still can be passed on to others.

When hepatitis A does produce symptoms, they may resemble those of flu or gastroenteritis in the beginning. There may be lassitude, weakness, loss of appetite, nausea, abdominal discomfort, fever, and headache. Often, the liver disease is distinguishable from flu by a loss of taste for smoking and a tender and aching liver, causing pain or pressure below the ribs of the right side. The urine also may be dark. After four to seven days, jaundice (yellow tint to whites of eyes and skin) may develop along with generalized itching, increased nausea and vomiting, the appearance of light-colored stools, and sometimes diarrhea. After another week or two, improvement begins but convalescence can be drawn out to weeks or months.

WHAT TO DO: There is no specific treatment for the virus. Bed rest is advisable when symptoms are at their height—and most patients will want to be in bed during that time. The diet should be well balanced, with adequate calories to avoid malnutrition. As symptoms begin to subside, bed rest is not essential.

Some physicians consider it possible to protect people in the family and others in close contact with a patient by injection of immune serum globulin, although effectiveness is not generally agreed upon by all medical authorities.

Hepatitis, Serum

This form of hepatitis is caused by a virus found in blood and tissues rather than in feces. It is spread by contaminated blood transfusions or when people, usually drug addicts, use the same contaminated needle and syringe.

The symptoms are much the same as for acute viral hepatitis. One difference is an outbreak of itching red wheals (hives) early in the course of the disease. In a minority of cases, there may also be a brief arthritis episode before jaundice appears.

WHAT TO DO: Treatment is the same as for acute viral hepatitis.

Hepatitis, Toxic

This is a liver inflammation caused by some drugs and chemicals (the latter often through occupational exposure). Prominent among causative agents are the dry-cleaning chemical carbon tetrachloride, insecticides, industrial solvents, and various metallic compounds, including those containing arsenic, gold, mercury, and iron. Drugs such as isoniazid, halothane anesthetic, bromates, chloral hydrate, potent tranquilizers, sulfa drugs, and some antibiotics may cause liver damage in people who are particularly sensitive to them.

Symptoms include nausea, vomiting, diarrhea, collapse, usually followed by jaundice, often with generalized itching, and sometimes by stupor and coma.

WHAT TO DO: Toxic hepatitis is serious. It can leave no aftermath, on the one hand; but on the other, it is capable of causing permanent injury or death.

The causative drug or chemical must be removed. Alcohol intake has to be banned. A high-protein, high-carbohydrate diet should be used.

Medical attention is advisable—and absolutely essential for anyone experiencing stupor or coma, in which case intravenous feeding as well as good nursing care will be required.

Hernia

If you have a bulge in your groin—in the right or left lower quadrant, or quarter, of the abdomen—or if your navel or belly button has started to protrude, chances are you have a hernia. It may, but does not always, give rise to abdominal pain.

Hernia is one of the most prevalent of human afflictions. With the exception of tonsillectomies, hernia repair operations are the most common, with about half a million done annually in the United States alone.

When a hernia acts up, there are measures you can take for relief; and there are guidelines, which I will give here, to indicate under what circumstances immediate surgery may be needed.

A hernia is a weak point in the abdominal wall through which a portion of intestine can protrude.

Around the abdominal organs lies the *peritoneum,* a thin, tough membrane that looks somewhat like Saran Wrap. It has a number of passageways through which certain structures pass in and out of the abdomen to go to other parts of the body: the femoral arteries that leave the larger arteries in the abdomen to supply blood to the legs; the spermatic cords that carry sperm cells from the testes into the abdomen and then to the penis; and the umbilical cord that emerges from the abdomen as an avenue for blood to nourish the fetus in the womb.

At any of these passageways, muscles and connective tissue that form the wall of the abdomen may weaken; and with the weakening, anything that adds to stress or strain on the abdomen—a sudden muscle pull, heavy lifting, coughing, straining at stool, marked weight gain, or pregnancy—may cause the intestine to press against the peritoneal lining and form a pouch which bulges out of the abdomen and is visible. This is a hernia.

A popular term for hernia is "rupture" which is inaccurate because it suggests tearing. Nothing is torn in a hernia.

TYPES OF HERNIA: The *inguinal* hernia occurs at the groin, in the anterior abdominal wall near where the thigh joins the trunk. It is the most common type, accounting for two thirds

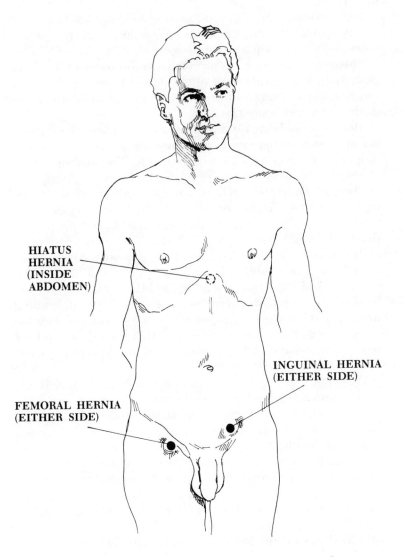

HIATUS
HERNIA
(INSIDE
ABDOMEN)

FEMORAL HERNIA
(EITHER SIDE)

INGUINAL HERNIA
(EITHER SIDE)

Fig. 23. Hernias: hiatus, femoral, inguinal

or more of all hernias, and is much more frequent in men than in women.

The *femoral* hernia occurs high up in the thigh and often can be felt about an inch or so below the groin. It is much more common in women than in men.

The *umbilical* hernia is a protrusion through the navel, or belly button. It occurs most often in infants, in which case it rarely requires surgery, but may also appear in adults, especially women after pregnancy.

An *incisional* hernia is a protrusion some time after a surgical operation at the site of the incision. It results from improper healing or excessive pressure on the healing tissue caused by straining, such as in lifting or severe coughing.

There is another type of hernia, not related to those discussed in this section—*hiatus* hernia—in which the stomach protrudes above the diaphragm through an enlarged opening in the diaphragm. This is treated separately in the next section.

RELIEVING A HERNIA YOURSELF: In the early stages, a hernia may be hardly noticeable, appearing as a soft lump under the skin, no bigger than a marble, and there may be no pain. In time, the lump size may increase. Often, the protruding intestinal section may slip out of the abdomen and into the hernial sac in the course of a day of activity and then slip back into normal position when you lie down. If it fails to slip back, you can often move it gently back.

To move it back, lie on your back with knees raised and gently push the lump back into the abdomen.

THE EMERGENCY SITUATION: If the lump fails to move back, you may be faced with an acute emergency requiring immediate medical attention.

It sometimes happens that as a hernia bulges out through a narrow opening (the neck), the intestine beyond the neck distends and becomes too large to return through the opening into the abdomen. A hernia caught in this manner is called *incarcerated* (imprisoned). If the neck is tight enough to cut off blood supply, the hernia swells further. This is a *strangulated* hernia. Unless blood supply is restored promptly, the intestine can become gangrenous, with potentially deadly consequences.

Pain and nausea may accompany a strangulated hernia, although occasionally, especially in older patients, there may be little or no pain.

SURGERY: Surgery can be lifesaving for a strangulated hernia. It can be curative, too, for an uncomplicated hernia. (Although a truss or abdominal support may be used for an uncomplicated hernia to hold the abdominal contents back, it may not be satisfactory and, of course, never cures the condition.)

In a hernia repair operation, the pushed-out loops of intestine are returned to the abdomen, the neck of the sac is tied, and the sac is then cut away. Muscle and fibrous tissue are overlapped to provide support, and if such support may not be fully adequate, a wire or plastic mesh may be stitched in for additional support. The mesh is strong but flexible enough so its presence afterward is not noticed.

Hernia repair can be carried out under general, spinal, or even local anesthesia. For a few days, there is some discomfort but usually not severe enough to require pain-killers. The patient is commonly up walking the day after surgery and home a few days later, the wound heals in about ten days, and normal strength in the abdominal wall is achieved in about six weeks, after which activities usually need not be limited. Although hernias sometimes recur, the improved surgical techniques now available provide a permanent cure rate of 90 percent.

SURGICAL AND NONSURGICAL TREATMENT FOR UMBILICAL HERNIA: Often, in infants, umbilical hernias heal themselves.

Actually, during fetal development in the womb, the intestine grows more rapidly than the abdominal cavity, and for a time part of the intestine lies outside the abdomen in a sac within the umbilical cord.

Usually by the time of birth the intestine is back in the abdomen, and the abdominal wall closes. Occasionally, however, the wall does not close solidly enough and a loop of intestine covered with skin protrudes, so that the navel of the child appears to be inflated. Actually, in most cases, there is no intestine in the protrusion but rather a fold of peritoneum called the omentum. The defect is more likely to occur in premature infants and in girls rather than boys.

Commonly, the abdominal wall defect closes by itself. Coughing, crying, and straining temporarily enlarge the sac, but the hernia never bursts and digestion is not affected. The hernia may be strapped with adhesive tape to aid healing and diminish the bulge.

If, however, an umbilical hernia has not repaired itself by the time a child is one or two years old, surgical repair can be carried out. Especially for a girl infant, repair may be advisable, since the hernia may enlarge later during pregnancy and require repair after delivery.

In the repair procedure, which may be done under general, spinal, or local anesthesia, the navel is lifted, the sac removed, the muscles brought together firmly, and the navel repositioned. Usually, in infants, no limitations are needed after the repair, but in adults activity may have to be limited for about six weeks until the repair is fully strengthened.

REPAIRING AN INCISIONAL HERNIA: When an incisional hernia occurs, a swelling about the incision or through it may become apparent, and there may be a hard lump that sometimes goes away when you lie down. Depending upon the site of the incision, the hernia may contain part of the intestine, stomach, or liver.

For repair, the incision is opened, the hernia sac removed, the muscle layers overlapped, and a plastic mesh may be inserted for additional support, after which the incision is stitched securely. Pain afterward is usually mild. You are likely to be up next day, home in a week or less.

Hernia, Hiatus

The *diaphragm*, a large flat muscle separating the chest from the abdomen, has openings through which pass blood vessels and nerves—and an opening, too, for the esophagus, or gullet, on its way to join the stomach. When the normal opening for the esophagus, called a *hiatus*, becomes enlarged, part of the stomach may push up into the chest, either inter-mittently or constantly. This is a hiatus hernia.

Often, the hernia produces no symptoms even though pres-ent for much of a lifetime. Commonly, it turns up during rou-tine chest x-rays in people totally without discomfort.

A hiatus hernia can cause severe pain when a pocket of air or fluid gets caught in the pouch of stomach lying in the chest. This is usually relieved by belching or the eventual passage of the air or fluid out of the pouch and into the lower stomach.

In some cases, the hernia may be associated with reflux of stomach acid into the esophagus, and pain results, which may range from mild heartburn to deep-seated ache behind the lower end of the breastbone. Sometimes the pain may radiate to the left shoulder, simulating the pain of a heart attack—but unlike a heart condition the pain does not increase with effort nor decrease with rest.

Typically, hiatus hernia pain begins almost immediately after meals, especially if there is any bending or lying down. It may be aggravated by a sneeze, cough, or straining at stool. Sleep may be interrupted by the pain.

WHAT TO DO: Sometimes, a few simple measures may suf-fice. One is to elevate the head of the bed six to eight inches on blocks to allow gravity to work for you during the night. If this causes you to slip downward in bed, it is equally effective to insert a board in top half of bed between mattress and springs, elevating the head of the bed about 45 degrees, simi-lar to a raised hospital bed. Elevating the head on pillows is useless, as there is a tendency to slip off them, and the upper part of the body is not satisfactorily raised.

Avoidance of tight belts or other tight items of clothing helps by avoiding the increased abdominal pressure they can produce, which can push the stomach through the hiatus opening into the chest.

When you have to bend down, do the bending at the knees rather than the waist as another means of avoiding increase of abdominal pressure and flow of stomach juices upward.

It can also be helpful in many cases to eat smaller meals more often, with the last no closer than two hours before bed-time.

For some people, reduction of the intake of carbonated drinks, coffee, and tea is useful. Smoking can be a factor, and its elimination, or at least reduction, can help.

Antacids may be of some use.

Surgery—to return the stomach to normal position and repair the hernia—can be used in severe cases that do not yield to simpler measures but should be looked upon as a last resort. It should be performed only by a specialty surgeon who regularly does such operations; otherwise the result may be worse than the original condition. Hiatus hernia repair is one of the most common operations to be performed unnecessarily; no specimen is removed to provide a means of determining whether the surgery was warranted.

Herpes Zoster (See SHINGLES)

Hiccup (Hiccough)

A hiccup or hiccough—*singultus*, in medical language—is an involuntary spasmodic contraction of the *diaphragm*, the flat muscle separating the chest and the abdomen, along with sudden closure of the *glottis*, the upper opening of the larynx, or voice box. The diaphragmatic contraction—actually, many contractions—leads to an urge to breathe in, but the glottis closes the airway so the air inflow is checked. And the peculiar noise of hiccups comes from the attempt to inhale while the air passage is closed.

Almost anything that can irritate or stimulate nerves or brain centers controlling diaphragmatic action and the action of other muscles of breathing can lead to hiccups. Among common causes are eating too fast, too much alcohol, swallowing hot, cold or irritating substances, and nervous tension. A bowel or other internal disorder may trigger hiccups. They sometimes follow surgery.

WHAT TO DO: Most hiccups are at worst annoying or embarrassing and soon stop or can be made to stop.

You can use the method that works best for you. It is a fact that a high level of carbon dioxide in the blood tends to stop hiccups. And you can increase the level by a series of breath-holdings or by rebreathing into a paper bag (not, however, a plastic bag, which can be dangerous).

Other home methods that may work: holding the tongue and pulling it forward; swallowing dry bread or crushed ice; sipping water slowly or, alternatively, swallowing it rapidly; applying a finger to each eye and gently massaging (never hard); swallowing a teaspoonful of dry sugar. It's not particularly pleasant but often hiccups can be stopped if you induce vomiting by sticking your finger into the back of your throat.

If hiccuping persists, it may be exhausting; occasionally it may indicate underlying disease. Medical help should be obtained. Almost always a physician can stop the hiccuping. Various sedative drugs and tranquilizers may be used. One simple method that very often is successful involves the introduction by the physician of a plastic or rubber suction tube through the nose to a distance of three or four inches to stimulate the pharynx by a jerky to-and-fro movement.

Hives and Giant Hives

In hives, which is also called *urticaria*, large red, raised patches (wheals) appear suddenly on the skin, accompanied by itching. The patches can range up to the size of a half dollar or sometimes even larger.

An outbreak can be caused by insect bites and jellyfish stings; by allergy to drugs or foods (among the most common: eggs, shellfish, nuts, fruits); or may follow some bacterial and viral infections.

Sometimes, the patches may come and go and, after remaining at one site for some hours, may disappear only to reappear elsewhere.

WHAT TO DO: Hives usually subside in one to seven days. If you know the cause and can avoid it, that is best. If the cause is not obvious and you are taking medication, any medication that your physician has told you is not essential should be stopped until the condition has disappeared.

If you have on hand an oral antihistamine drug—such as cyproheptadine or diphenhydramine—check with your physician by phone about using it. It often can relieve symptoms.

Giant Hives

Giant hives, a more serious form of hives which is also known as *angioneurotic edema* or *angioedema*, appears as large swellings on the lips, tongue, eyelids, genitalia, or other parts of the body.

Giant hives can be an emergency situation calling for immediate medical help when, on rare occasions, the airway is affected, leading to breathing distress and asthmalike wheezing. In such cases, an injection of epinephrine is needed, and this may be supplemented with nebulized epinephrine applied by spray. Such treatment usually will prevent airway obstruction. In rare cases, a throat incision to permit breathing may be required, and oxygen too may be administered.

If no medical help is at hand, give an antihistamine—any "cold" or hay fever pill. If the person can breathe in but not out, use the Heimlich maneuver (see p. 44) to get air out of the lungs. Use the maneuver after each inhalation until exhaling occurs naturally.

Hoarseness

Hoarseness stems from irritation of the vocal cords. One common cause is the common cold. Another, especially when the hoarseness is mild, is cigarette smoke. An episode of hoarseness may also indicate acute inflammation of the larynx (see LARYNGITIS). In children, prolonged yelling or screaming can lead to hoarseness.

WHAT TO DO: Hoarseness is not easy to overcome. It takes time for the irritated area to heal.

Some measures are helpful. Rest the voice as much as possible. If you're a smoker, try to stop smoking to help the healing process. Adding moisture to the air with a humidifier or vaporizer and increasing your fluid intake are valuable measures.

If the hoarseness persists, lasting for more than two or three weeks after a cold or other respiratory infection has passed and you have stopped smoking, it then should have medical investigation.

Rarely, cancer may cause persistent hoarseness. Much more common causes are polyps or cysts in the vocal cords.

Hookworm (See WORM-INDUCED DISEASES)

Hyperventilation (See OVERBREATHING)

Hypoglycemia (Low Blood Sugar)

Hypoglycemia, a condition in which blood sugar falls to abnormally low levels, can be manifested by diverse symptoms several hours after meals.

The symptoms may include one or more of the following: flushing or pallor, chilliness, numbness, hunger, trembling, headache, dizziness, weakness, palpitation, faintness, convulsions.

Glucose (blood sugar) provides ready energy for all body tissues and is especially vital to the brain, which depends upon it almost entirely for energy needs. Normally, the blood glucose level is in a fairly constant range between 60 and 100 milligrams per 100 milliliters. When carbohydrates are consumed, they are converted into glucose, and any excess of the sugar goes to the liver for storage as *glycogen*. As tissues use glucose, lowering the blood sugar level, glycogen is reconverted to glucose and moves into the blood. If glucose is insufficient, other materials in the liver are turned into the sugar.

One cause of hypoglycemia is an excess of insulin. The excess may result from an overdose in a diabetic or from a rare insulin-secreting tumor of the pancreas. Another possible cause is insufficiency of certain hormones needed to counteract insulin; this may stem from a pituitary or adrenal gland deficiency.

Hypoglycemia may occur in some children who happen to be sensitive to fructose (a sugar found in large amounts in fruits and honey) or to galactose (a material in milk), or who have inadequate enzymes needed to produce glucose from glycogen. These are familial disorders which often become less of a problem as the child grows.

Most often in adults, however, there is no known cause and the hypoglycemia is called functional.

WHAT TO DO: If you suffer an episode of symptoms that might be due to hypoglycemia, they can usually be relieved promptly with some orange juice, candy, or honey.

For more certain diagnosis, a physician can measure the blood glucose level after you drink a solution of glucose.

In functional hypoglycemia, attacks usually can be avoided by a high-protein, low-carbohydrate diet with a snack on waking and another on retiring. If diet alone fails, small doses of corticosteroids may help.

Other forms of hypoglycemia, of course, require different treatment. Surgical removal is curative if there is a pancreatic tumor. In pituitary or adrenal gland insufficiency, treatment with adrenal steroid hormone may be needed. If sensitivity to fructose or galactose is the problem, foods containing the material should be avoided.

Hysteria

This is a state of tension or excitement in which control over the emotions is lost temporarily. It can be brought on by danger, severe fright, bad news, or any incident that pushes a person beyond normal endurance and, for the moment, seems unbearable.

There may be such symptoms as wild crying or shouting, pointless laughter, aimless walking about, or a temper tantrum.

WHAT TO DO: Usually, such a hysterical outburst ends in a short time. When it does not, some cold water thrown into the face or a few light slaps may help.

Occasionally, fainting may occur. Use the simple measures for fainting noted at FAINTNESS AND FAINTING.

Impetigo

A highly contagious skin infection, usually caused by strep bacteria, impetigo is a disease of infants and young children, occurring only rarely in adults.

It produces pustules (pus-filled lesions) that rupture or crust within a few hours to several days. The crusted-over sores tend to be characteristic of the disease.

Arms, legs, and face tend to be more susceptible to impetigo than unexposed body areas. The disease may follow insect bites, fungal and other skin infections, but also can develop on normal healthy skin.

WHAT TO DO: This is a disease that requires medical help. Neglected impetigo can persist for months and may cause loss of skin pigmentation, sometimes with scarring. Sometimes, too, untreated impetigo may spread to deeper tissues.

While you may elect to try an antibiotic ointment if you have one on hand, prompt and effective control of impetigo usually requires a suitable antibiotic taken by mouth, which your physician can prescribe.

Indigestion (Dyspepsia)

Also called *upset stomach*, indigestion is not a specific ailment but rather a class of symptoms which can be varied in nature.

There may be a sense of discomfort in the abdomen. Nausea, heartburn, upper abdominal pain, a sense of fullness, a feeling of abdominal distention, gas, and belching may occur singly or in combination.

The possible causes are many: gallbladder disease, liver disease, peptic ulcer, intestinal obstruction, appendicitis, food poisoning, intolerance for milk or another food.

But in the vast majority of episodes of indigestion—and few of us escape an occasional bout—the common causes are eating too much or too rapidly, inadequate chewing, eating during emotional upsets, and swallowing large amounts of air. Other factors are excessive smoking, constipation, eating foods with excessively high fat content—and, in some cases, eating radishes, cucumbers, beans, cabbage, turnips, onions, and possibly such seasonings as chili, garlic, and pepper.

If you fail to chew food thoroughly, the stomach may secrete more acid in its digestive efforts—and the extra acid, in combination with excessive air that may enter the stomach because of hurried chewing and swallowing, may irritate the stomach lining.

Many symptoms of indigestion result from altered stomach motor activity. Normally, stomach *motility*—its useful churning activity—is stimulated when the stomach is moderately distended with food. But marked distention, as from overeating, may inhibit the activity and produce nausea as well as a sense of fullness.

Emotional upsets such as fear or depression tend to slow stomach activity. So may pain anywhere in the body or physical fatigue.

Alcohol and coffee may overly increase stomach activity. Smoking may decrease it and delay stomach emptying. Constipation may contribute to indigestion by distending the rectum and causing unusual awareness and concern over what is going on in the gastrointestinal tract.

WHAT TO DO: Although many people rush immediately to take antacids or other medication for indigestion, very often symptoms disappear if nothing more is done than to refrain from eating for several hours.

And you can sometimes relieve indigestion by loosening

any tight-fitting clothes and by lying down—*but* lie down on your right side. On the right side, you allow gravity to help the stomach move its contents along to the intestine.

To avoid stomach upsets, it helps greatly to eat a normal, balanced diet, in moderate amounts, without haste, in a relaxing atmosphere, and to avoid smoking beforehand.

If you experience frequent mild upsets, it can be useful to keep a diary of the food you eat to see if you can detect a pattern relating upsets with certain foods. If you find one or more culprits, avoid them.

If constipation is a factor, increased physical activity may help, and getting more fiber in your diet is very likely to be of value. You can get the fiber through fruits and vegetables, by using bread made with whole-grain rather than highly refined white flour, and by using a bran cereal or by adding unprocessed bran to your other cereals, sprinkling on a few table-spoonsful. Sometimes constipation is caused simply by not drinking enough fluids.

If excessive air swallowing is a factor, see AIR SWALLOWING for suggestions.

When indigestion is chronic, the possibility that it may be related to disease should be investigated by a physician.

Influenza (Flu)

A severe but usually relatively brief respiratory infection, influenza is caused by three groups of viruses, called A (which includes Asian flu), B, and C. Each group has variant viruses but all produce similar symptoms that vary only in intensity.

Spread by droplets from sneezes and coughs, influenza is highly contagious, with an incubation period of about 48 hours before symptoms appear.

The first symptoms, which often develop suddenly, are chilliness and fever up to 102° or 103°F. Other early symptoms include prostration and generalized aches and pains, which are most pronounced in the back and legs. Headache is common and is often accompanied by sensitivity to light. Respiratory symptoms—sore throat, burning below the breastbone, nonproductive cough, and sometimes nasal discharge—may be mild at first but later may become more pronounced.

Usually, after two or three days, symptoms begin to subside rapidly and fever is over (but sometimes fever may last as long as five days without complications). Fatigue, weakness, and excessive sweating may persist for several days or sometimes several weeks after other symptoms are gone.

WHAT TO DO: During the stage of acute symptoms and for 24 to 48 hours after temperature drops to normal, adequate rest—preferably bed rest—and avoidance of exertion are indicated.

For fever and discomfort, one or two 5-grain tablets of aspirin every four hours can be taken. If nasal obstruction is severe, one or two drops of 0.25 percent phenylephrine (as in Neo-Synephrine, for example) instilled into the nose often help. Excessive use of the drops, however, should be avoided, since that may cause a rebound reaction and increased stuffiness. Warm salt-water gargles are helpful for sore throat. Steam inhalation is often very useful in relieving respiratory symptoms.

Special note: There is a drug, amantadine hydrochloride, which your physician may prescribe for influenza. It is often used for shaking palsy (parkinsonism), but it also has been found to have some usefulness for influenza. Amantadine appears to be antiviral in this sense: it has no direct effect on flu viruses themselves but rather acts to decrease their penetration into body cells where they can multiply.

When there is an epidemic of flu of severe type, the physician may prescribe amantadine early in the disease when it may sometimes considerably alleviate symptoms. The drug also can be prescribed for preventive purposes for family members and others in close contact with the sick one and, generally, for people at high risk because of age or chronic health problems.

INFLUENZA COMPLICATIONS: It is possible for bacterial infection to occur as a complication when flu weakens body defenses. The risk is greater for the elderly and chronically ill.

Bacterial infection of the breathing tubes and sometimes

pneumonia may be indicated when fever, cough, and other respiratory symptoms last beyond five days.

Pneumonia should be suspected if you experience breathing difficulty, blueness, coughing up of blood, a new rise in temperature, or a relapse. With pneumonia, coughing will increase and produce bloody sputum.

If you experience any of the indications of possible complications, call a physician without delay so that suitable antibiotic treatment can be started to bring the complications under control and achieve cure, which is almost always possible.

Insect and Other Bug Bites and Stings

Stings by Hymenoptera (Yellow Jackets, Bees, Hornets, Wasps)

These are among the most painful and common insect stings. For some people who are specially sensitive, they can be deadly unless precautions are taken.

In stinging, insects of the order Hymenoptera inject venom under the skin. Normally, the venom produces a few minutes of fierce burning followed by reddening and itching at the site. A welt may form and subside in 3 or 4 hours. Most traces of the sting may be gone in about 24 hours.

WHAT TO DO: Stinger and venom, if they remain in the wound, should be scraped out with a fingernail or knife blade. Before and after they are removed, wash with soap and water.

Simple remedies then usually suffice. If you have it available, sprinkle some ordinary household meat tenderizer on a square of gauze or a handkerchief and apply for 20 to 30 minutes. If tenderizer is not available, an ice pack or cold compresses can be applied, and calamine or another soothing lotion dabbed on. For persistent itching, some people find it helpful to apply a baking powder–ammonia paste, made by mixing baking powder and ordinary household cleaning ammonia. Antihistamine tablets, if available, help relieve itching. So may aspirin.

SERIOUS REACTIONS: In a person sensitive to the venom, the reaction to a sting is another matter—not local but systemic, or generalized.

Even a mild systemic reaction—with generalized hives, itching, malaise, and anxiety—is to be taken seriously, since it can indicate that the next sting may produce more serious, even life-threatening consequences.

In the more serious reaction, anaphylactic shock occurs. This is a combination of symptoms and signs that may include

Labored breathing	Weakness
Swallowing difficulty	Blueness
Chest constriction	Rapid fall in blood pressure
Abdominal pain	Collapse
Nausea	Incontinence
Vomiting	Unconsciousness
Confusion	

Note: Some people experience delayed reactions. Not until 10 to 14 days after a sting do they develop symptoms of fever, gland swelling, headache, hives, joint pains, and malaise. If they are stung again, the next response may be immediate and severe.

WHO DEVELOPS SEVERE REACTIONS: There is an increased tendency for people with other allergies—such as hay fever, asthma, or drug sensitivities—or who come from families with histories of such allergies to be sensitive to insect venom. People over the age of 30 seem more prone than younger people but that does not mean that the young are exempt.

But anyone who notices that the reaction at the site worsens with each succeeding sting is getting a warning that a serious reaction may be ahead. Skin tests with insect extract may then verify the sensitivity.

WHAT TO DO: When a severe reaction occurs, immediate treatment is essential. Death can occur within 10 to 15 minutes after a sting in some cases.

The key element in treatment is an under-the-skin injection of epinephrine (Adrenalin), with vigorous massage of the injection site to speed absorption. In some cases, a second injec-

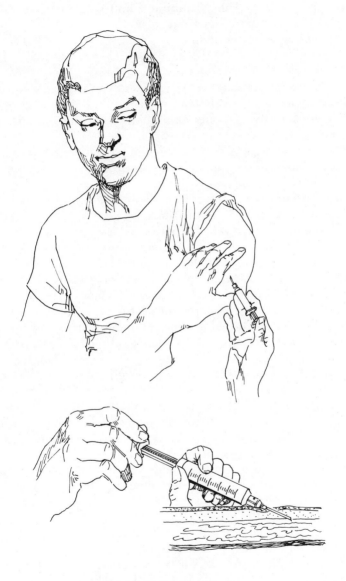

Fig. 24. Subcutaneous injection.

tion may be needed in 20 minutes, and sometimes several repetitions. Antihistamine may also be administered, and other measures may be required.

With such care, there is usually quick recovery, and the victim may be discharged within a few hours.

But professional emergency treatment is not always immediately available. For this reason, many physicians now prescribe, for sensitive patients, a lifesaving sting kit to be carried whenever they may be exposed to insects.

The kit contains a syringe preloaded with epinephrine, along with antihistamine tablets, sterilizing swabs, tourniquet, and instructions.

After use of the kit, the patient should be seen by a physician, but the kit buys valuable time.

Not only anyone who has experienced a severe generalized reaction but anyone with increasingly severe local reactions should consider injections to build tolerance. The injections begin with low concentrations of insect body extracts which are gradually increased until sufficient tolerance is built up to withstand any reasonable amount of stinging. Thereafter, tolerance is maintained by injections at monthly or longer intervals. Each visit to a physician's office or clinic for an injection can be very brief.

Desensitization, as the injection procedure is called, is not 100 percent effective but does confer a significant degree of protection in the great majority of those who receive it. Now under investigation are injections using pure venom instead of insect body extracts. The pure venom gives promise of providing even more effective desensitization.

AVOIDING STINGS: Certain guidelines for minimizing the likelihood of Hymenoptera stings should be heeded not only by the sensitive but also by those not yet sensitive—for the fewer the stings, the less likelihood of developing serious insect allergy:

1. With appropriate precaution, destroy any Hymenoptera nests around the house or yard. Most often, you find wasps nesting under eaves and windowsills. The nests can be knocked down with a broom handle. Yellow jackets commonly nest in old stumps and holes in the ground. They can often be

discouraged with kerosene, gasoline, or lye applied at night when they are home. No fires are needed; the fumes do the work.

2. Wear shoes and socks outdoors. And to avoid seeming like a flower to insects, eschew scented soaps, lotions, shampoos, perfumes. Also avoid floral prints and bright colors. And don't wear floppy clothes that can entangle and infuriate insects.

3. Be wary about garbage cans, which often attract insects. Also attractive to Hymenoptera: melting ice cream cones and watermelon. Make it a practice at picnics to keep food covered until served; quickly pack away leftovers.

4. Don't try to swat an insect that may sting. Move away slowly. If retreat is impossible, lie face down, with arms covering the head. If an insect should get into your car, stop and carefully open the windows and doors so the insect may fly out. Or, moving slowly and warily, get yourself out. It's a good idea for the specially sensitive to keep a spray can of insecticide handy in the car in season.

5. Possibly helpful: vitamin B $_1$ (thiamine)—100 milligrams for an adult, 50 for a child—on a day when you may be exposed to insects. The vitamin is excreted in perspiration and the smell may repel insects.

Tick Bites

Measuring from one fourth to three fourths of an inch when mature, ticks are gray or brown oval insects with small heads. They are found in all parts of the United States, on low shrubs, grass, and trees. Ticks sometimes carry disease such as Rocky Mountain spotted fever, tularemia, and Colorado tick fever. In rare cases, in children and small adults, they produce paralysis, which is quickly overcome once the tick is removed.

WHAT TO DO: A tick attaches itself to the skin and sucks blood. It's important to remove rather than kill it.

To remove, cover the insect with a heavy oil (such as mineral, salad, or machine oil). The oil closes the insect's breathing pores and it may release its hold immediately; if not, allow the oil to remain for half an hour. Then carefully remove the tick with tweezers, making sure that all parts come out.

Oil appears to be the best method of removal but other methods may be used. They include applying a heated needle or lighted cigarette to the tick's body, then using tweezers. There is some risk with the latter methods of injury to the skin and of leaving some tick parts in the wound.

Once the tick is removed, gently but thoroughly give the site a soap-and-water scrub. An antiseptic may be applied.

Chiggers

Very tiny—about one-twentieth of an inch long—a chigger is an oval bug, usually with red velvety coloring but sometimes colorless. The adult, which is harmless, has eight legs and resembles a small spider. The culprit larva has six legs. Chiggers are found in low damp places covered with vegetation such as shaded woods, high grass or weeds, fruit orchards, and lawns and golf courses.

A chigger larva attaches itself to the skin by sticking its mouthparts into the follicle of a hair. It then injects enzymes that help it feed on human cells; it does not suck blood. Several hours later, intense itching results from the enzymes and small red welts appear.

WHAT TO DO: To remove chiggers, lather with soap and rinse several times. Cold packs or a towel dipped in ice water may help relieve symptoms.

Spiders

Spiders in the United States are generally harmless, with the exception of the black widow and the brown recluse.

BLACK WIDOW: The black widow is not difficult to identify. It has a dark brown to glossy black body about a quarter of an inch wide and one and a half inches long overall with legs extended. The female, which is poisonous, has a red or yellow hourglass marking on the underside of the abdomen; the non-poisonous male does not have this. The black widow is found throughout the United States and southern Canada in outdoor sheds and privies, under stones and logs, in hollow stumps and brush piles, and sometimes indoors in dark corners of garages, barns, and piles of wood.

A black widow bite causes local redness, and two tiny red spots may appear. Almost immediately there is sharp pain, which may go away. In about 30 minutes, the venom causes the abdominal muscles to become rigid. Later there may be great pain in the limbs and difficulty in breathing and talking. A black widow bite may cause death from breathing paralysis in about 5 percent of cases and is more dangerous for children.

What to Do for a Black Widow Bite: The victim should be taken as quickly as possible to a physician or emergency room, since medical care and a serum will be needed. In transporting, try to keep the victim as calm and quiet as possible. If available, apply an antiseptic such as alcohol or hydrogen peroxide to the bitten area to help prevent secondary infection. Pack ice around the bite to slow spread of the venom.

BROWN RECLUSE: Found in southern and midwestern United States, this spider gets its name because it prefers dark places where it is seldom disturbed—outside in old trash piles and debris, indoors in attics, closets, dresser drawers, the other dark areas. It has an oval, light yellow to dark brown body, three-eighths to one-fourth inch long, a quarter of an inch wide, with eight legs and distinctive fiddle-shaped mark on its back.

Left alone, the brown recluse is shy and will not bite. When it does bite, the sting is almost painless at first. In two to eight hours, there may be pain followed by blisters, swelling, or ulceration—and, in some cases, rash, nausea, jaundice, chills, fever, cramps, or joint pain.

What to Do: Pack ice around the bite and call a physician. Antihistamines and cortisonelike drugs help to keep the sore area from spreading and also help promote healing. Without quick medical action, weak adults and children have been known to die from a brown recluse bite.

Scorpions

Present in most of the United States, scorpions are not all dangerous. Those that are occur only in the Southwest. These creatures have a crablike appearance with clawlike pincers and a fleshy five-segment tail ending in a bulbous sac or stinger. About two and one-fourth to four inches in size, the two poisonous types are solid straw yellow or yellow with irregular black stripes on their back. By day, they are found under stones, bark, boards, outhouse floors and burrowing in sand. At night they roam, crawl under doors into houses.

Scorpions sting by thrusting their tail overhead. Swelling or discoloration of the stung area usually means a painful but *not dangerous* bite. A *dangerous* poisonous sting usually does not change the appearance of the area, which does, however, become very sensitive. With a poisonous sting, facial contortions may follow and much saliva flow. A fever of 104°F or more develops, the tongue becomes sluggish, and there may be increasingly intense convulsions, which may be fatal.

WHAT TO DO: The first few hours are critical. Keep the victim quiet, call a physician immediately, apply a tourniquet if possible between the sting site and the heart. Do not give pain-killers, which may increase the toxicity of the venom. Use of antitoxin by a physician is very effective.

Tarantulas

These dark spiders have a furry covering and are quite large (six to seven inches in diameter, toe to toe). Tarantulas are found in the southwestern part of the United States and the tropics. Only the tropical varieties are poisonous. A tarantula will not bite unless teased, and the bite produces a negligible pinprick sensation.

WHAT TO DO: Wash and apply antiseptic to prevent possible secondary infection.

Bedbugs

From one-eighth to one-fourth inch long, with flat oval body, short broad head, and six legs, and with an unpleasant, pungent odor, a bedbug adult is reddish brown while the young is yellowish white.

Bedbugs hide in crevices, mattresses, or under loose wallpaper by day. At night, they travel some distance to find victims.

A bedbug punctures the skin and sucks blood. While feeding, it secretes an enzyme that produces local inflammation and welts. Different people are affected differently. Some aren't bothered; others have marked swelling and irritation. A bug usually bites a sleeping victim, gorges for up to about five minutes, then departs, so it is rarely necessary to remove one.

WHAT TO DO: Apply antiseptic to prevent possible infection. When bedbugs are found, there is usually a large group of them living together. Spray beds, mattresses, bedsprings, and baseboards with insecticide.

Insomnia

Few of us escape an occasional episode of difficulty in falling or staying asleep. Occasional insomnia, however annoying, is likely to be of little medical importance. Chronic sleeping problems, however, deserve medical investigation, perhaps by experts in one of the sleep laboratories now to be found in more and more medical centers.

Sometimes, the occasional episode of insomnia—or even what seems to be chronic insomnia—is not insomnia at all. There is no such thing as an "ideal" or "normal" amount of sleep. The needed amount varies considerably. If you can work and play through the day without feeling exhausted or irritable, you probably had sufficient sleep the night before—even if the amount seemed less than adequate. The fact is that some people who may think they need and try to get seven and a half to eight hours or even more sleep nightly simply do not require that much.

WHAT TO DO: Many factors over which you may have some control can interfere with sleep. Perhaps too much light is getting into the room; try eyeshades. If too much noise, earplugs may help. A change of mattress sometimes can be a major contribution to better sleep.

Not only coffee and tea but various soft drinks contain caffeine which, if taken late in the day, may interfere with sleep for some people. Some drugs, including some of the appetite suppressants, contain stimulant agents.

There are many home remedies which work for some people. One, warm milk at bedtime, recently has been found to have a scientific basis. L-tryptophan, which occurs in milk, is a natural amino acid, a building block of protein. In sleep laboratory studies, L-tryptophan has been found to make for drowsiness and to be capable of halving the fall-asleep time for many people. Other home remedies include warm baths, bad books, old TV movies, soft music, and aspirin.

Several drugs available without prescription are supposed to have sleep-inducing properties. Usually they contain antihistamines, with a sedating side effect. They are mild, may occasionally be helpful, but are not likely to solve any problems of chronic insomnia.

Prescription drugs for sleep may help on occasion, during a time of special stress. But if used often, they lose their effectiveness even as they often become habit-forming, making the situation worse. So stay away from chronic use of "sleeping pills" and, instead, find out what is causing your sleep problem.

One new approach to chronic insomnia is worth noting because it provides a method you can try. It is concerned with the relationship between insomnia and bad sleeping habits and how to correct the habits.

A leading researcher in this area is Dr. Richard R. Bootzin, a Northwestern University psychologist, who considers misuse of the bed to be an especially pernicious habit.

To overcome it, Dr. Bootzin gives patients specific instructions, which are illustrated in the case of a young man who for four years had gone to bed nightly at midnight and been unable to fall asleep until three or four in the morning, stewing about various problems and often resorting to TV to try to stop stewing.

Bootzin's instructions to him: Go to bed only when tired, and once in the bedroom—no TV watching, reading, or worrying. Stay in bed to sleep, not to stew. If sleep doesn't come within a short time, leave the bed and the room. Return to bed only when you're ready to try to fall asleep again. If you still don't succeed soon, get out of bed and room again, repeating the process until you do get to sleep quickly after getting back to bed. No matter whether it is a weekday or weekend, and no matter how much sleep you get in a night, set the alarm for the same time every morning. The body needs rest, and a regular schedule will help you get it.

Typically, Dr. Bootzin has reported, the patient in this case at first had to leave the bedroom four and five times a night. But after two weeks of increasingly associating the bedroom with sleep rather than worry, reading, or TV, he was getting two to four hours more sleep each night and, at the end of two months, was leaving the bedroom no more than once a week.

If you wake several hours after falling asleep and have difficulty getting back to sleep, it is better, I have found, not to fight the problem. Get up, eat a light snack, do something constructive until you feel ready for sleep again.

Insulin Shock (See DIABETIC REACTIONS)

Intertrigo (See CHAFING)

Intestinal Obstruction

Obstruction, which interferes with normal passage of intestinal contents, may occur in either the small or large bowel and may be either partial or complete.

Symptoms vary with the site and degree of obstruction.

Complete small intestine obstruction: With this, there is severe, on-off, cramplike pain around the navel area, and vomiting soon follows. Vomiting and pain at first coincide. Later vomiting occurs irregularly and may include fecal matter in the vomitus. If the obstruction is high up in the small intestine, there is little abdominal distention; if low, distention is conspicuous. Once any retained gas below the obstruction is passed, gas no longer is expelled from the rectum.

Partial small intestine obstruction: Symptoms are similar to those of complete small intestine obstruction but less severe, and cramps may be followed by diarrhea. Partial obstruction may recur on a chronic basis, clearing itself spontaneously, or, on the other hand, it may progress to complete obstruction.

Complete colon (large bowel) obstruction: Symptoms often develop insidiously. Slowly the abdomen becomes distended. Vomiting is infrequent. Pain occurs but is less severe than in small intestine obstruction. No gas is passed from the rectum.

Partial colon obstruction: Symptoms are similar to complete colon obstruction. There are on-off abdominal cramps and constipation; in some cases, constipation and diarrhea may alternate.

CAUSES: One cause is an adhesion. The normal bowel is coiled somewhat like a hose, and the loops of intestine move smoothly over each other. As the result of infection or injury, sometimes stemming from an old operation, an area of loop surface may become dry, and scarlike tissue may develop. That area then may adhere to other tissue, including another intestinal loop. This is an adhesion—and with it there may be twisting and knotting, leading to obstruction.

Another cause of obstruction is an inguinal (groin) hernia, which may allow a loop of intestine to get caught in it.

Adhesions and hernias are the most common causes of mechanical obstruction.

A less common cause is volvulus. This is a condition in which a loop of intestine twists on itself; and the tissue (mesentery) that attaches the intestine to the back wall of the abdomen, and carries its blood supply, also becomes twisted. Just as you can stop the flow of water by tightly twisting a garden hose, so with a twisted intestine, nothing can pass; it is obstructed. The twisted mesentery cuts off the bowel's blood supply. Volvulus is more common in older people than younger.

Intussusception, another less common cause, mostly affects children under the age of three. In this condition, one part of the small intestine telescopes into the colon and cannot withdraw, like a Chinese finger puzzle, and obstruction results.

Another possible cause is cancer.

WHAT TO DO: If you suspect an intestinal obstruction of any kind, get medical help quickly. Delay can lead to gangrene of the bowel, peritonitis, and death.

Plain x-ray films of the abdomen often aid diagnosis by showing dilated loops of intestine indicative of obstruction. X-ray films taken after a barium enema may be used to point to obstruction in the colon.

The aim of treatment is to overcome the obstruction as quickly as possible while supporting the patient with fluids by vein and pain-relieving agents.

For an incomplete obstruction, a long tube is inserted through the nose into the intestine, and sometimes is effective in relieving the blockage. If not, surgery is undertaken without delay. When obstruction is complete, surgery is done on an emergency basis to prevent development of a dangerous toxic state, possible rupture of the distended intestine followed by peritonitis, or strangulation as blood supply is cut off, leading to gangrene within a few hours.

When obstruction stems from adhesions, surgery may involve only simple cutting of the adhesions. For a hernia-caused obstruction, the bowel segment is freed from the hernial sac and dropped back into the abdominal cavity. In volvulus, the intestinal loop can be straightened during surgery and attached to the side of the abdominal cavity.

In a child with intussusception, a telescoped loop of intestine sometimes may slip free of its own accord. Sometimes, too, a barium enema being used for diagnosis may cause it to slip free. In most cases, the loop can be readily freed and restored to normal position by surgery.

When the intestine is cancerous or gangrenous, the diseased section must be removed and the two healthy ends attached to restore continuity. Large segments of intestine can be removed without interfering with normal function.

Reassuringly, the success rate for intestinal obstruction surgery is high—about 91 percent even though there is often some delay on the part of the patient seeking help. The success rate is likely to improve further with early diagnosis and operation.

"Itch, The" (See SCABIES)

Itching

Itching, known medically as *pruritus*, has a great variety of possible causes. It may accompany various skin diseases such as hives, eczema, contact dermatitis (allergic reaction to materials contacting the skin), insect bites, prickly heat (see MIL-IARIA), and scabies (see SCABIES).

Dry skin, especially in older people, can cause generalized itching. In some women during the later months of pregnancy, itching may occur without any skin lesions. Many drugs, including barbiturates (sleeping pills), can cause itching.

Generalized itching can accompany some internal diseases, and sometimes may be the only troublesome symptom. Among such diseases are gallbladder disease and uremia (often associated with hyperparathyroidism, or excessive functioning of the parathyroid glands in the neck area).

WHAT TO DO: Scratching does not really help, although it may seem to relieve discomfort briefly. Actually, scratching may lower the itch threshold and bring on a cycle of itch–scratch–more-itch–more-scratch. It can also cause additional discomfort if the skin is broken.

When itching is generalized and persistent, medical help may be needed to determine and treat the cause.

If possible, all medication should be stopped on the chance a medication may be involved. Woolen or other irritating clothing should be avoided. Bathing should be kept to a minimum, since it may aggravate generalized itching from any cause. A lukewarm bath with cornstarch sprinkled into it, however, may give temporary relief. Applying a white petrolatum, particularly one containing 0.125 to 0.25 percent menthol, can be soothing.

Anal Itching

The area about the anus is particularly susceptible to a scratch-itch cycle, since the skin is almost always moist and is exposed to fecal matter.

Possible causes of anal itching include poor hygiene, minor

injuries produced by defecation, irritating soaps and clothing, local disease such as hemorrhoids, infectious agents, intestinal parasites such as pinworms, allergic reactions, and systemic disorders such as jaundice, diabetes, uremia, and lymphoma.

Otherwise inexplicable itching, recent research suggests, may be caused by any of six common dietary items—coffee, tea, cola, beer, chocolate, and tomatoes. Such itching occurs 24 to 48 hours after a certain "threshold" amount (for a sensitive person) of one or more of the items is consumed. For example, the average threshold for a person sensitive to coffee seems to be two and a half cups a day, with three cups causing itching and two not doing so.

WHAT TO DO: To help relieve anal itching until a cause can be found, scratching must be stopped, however difficult to do so. Keep the skin in the area clean and dry. Apply talc or dusting powder often, after thoroughly drying the skin with tissue or cotton. If necessary, your physician can prescribe a corticosteroid preparation such as triamcinolone acetonide to be applied two or three times a day; it usually provides relief.

Jaundice (See GALLBLADDER DISEASE; HEPATITIS)

Jock Itch (See RINGWORM INFECTIONS)

Joint Pain (See GOUT; MUSCLE AND JOINT PAIN, TENDERNESS, STIFFNESS)

Kidney Infection (See URINARY TRACT INFECTIONS)

Kidney Stone

The passage of a kidney stone can produce one of the most excruciating of all pains.

Stones vary in size, all the way from those no larger than grains of sand to some that are an inch or more in diameter. Not uncommonly, they can be present in some numbers in the kidney without producing any trouble; these are the so-called silent stones.

But when a stone, usually of larger size, obstructs the *ureter*, the tube connecting the kidney to the bladder, *renal colic* results. Typical symptoms include agonizing on-off pain, usu-

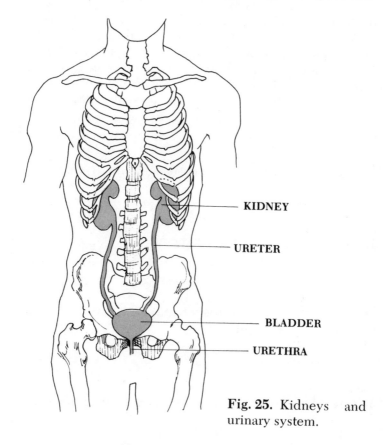

KIDNEY

URETER

BLADDER

URETHRA

Fig. 25. Kidneys and urinary system.

ally starting in the flank (the side of the body between ribs and hip) or kidney area (toward the back of the abdomen at about the level of the lowest ribs), and spreading across the abdomen often into the area of the genitalia and inner side of the thigh.

Nausea, vomiting, and abdominal distention may be present along with chills and fever. A need to urinate frequently may be felt. Blood may appear in the urine.

WHAT TO DO: Get medical attention as quickly as possible. You will need it, first of all, for the pain, which is likely to be controllable with nothing less than morphine or meperidine.

Sometimes, during an attack, a stone will work its way out of the body spontaneously, passing through the ureter into the bladder and then through the urethra to be expelled with urine.

You may be given large quantities of fluids—as much as three or more quarts per day—along with antispasmodic medication to encourage the stone to pass if it does not do so spontaneously.

If the stone still fails to pass and continues to obstruct, surgery may be required to prevent or overcome complications. A kidney stone, if it blocks passage of urine, can cause backpressure and infection and may eventually lead to kidney destruction.

If a stone happens to be lodged toward the lower end of the ureter, it may sometimes be removed with the aid of a *cystoscope*. The instrument is passed into the bladder, and a long, thin, loop-tipped catheter is moved through the scope into the ureter. With the loop, it may be possible to maneuver the stone into the bladder where it can be removed through the scope. Stones too firmly lodged to be removed in this way can be removed through an open operation, with an incision in the abdomen or back over the stone area. About 200,000 kidney stone operations are performed yearly in this country.

PREVENTING RECURRENCES: The passage of one stone does not by any means preclude future trouble from other stones. Preventive efforts are important and require medical help.

Stones are of various types, and once one is passed or removed, it should be analyzed to determine its nature.

Many stones are composed of *calcium*. They occur in people who secrete large amounts of calcium in the urine. One cause for such secretion is *hyperparathyroidism*—overactivity of the parathyroid glands (four small bodies attached to the thyroid gland in the neck). The parathyroids secrete *parathormone*, a hormone involved in regulating the balance in the body of calcium derived from milk and other foods and its excretion in the urine. If the parathyroids secrete too much hormone, excessive amounts of calcium are excreted. For this, parathyroid surgery is effective.

In some cases, calcium stones are formed in the absence of a gland problem—because more than usual amounts of calcium are absorbed from the diet or drinking water. Often, stone formation can be prevented by reducing intake of dairy foods, the main source of dietary calcium. If diet change is not enough, a thiazide diuretic ("water pill") can be used.

Uric acid stones are another type. People who develop such stones have excess uric acid in their blood. They may or may not have gout, with which high uric acid levels are commonly associated. But the more uric acid in the blood, the more that has to be eliminated through the kidneys; some of the uric acid not washed away with urine forms crystals, which become the basis for stones. Uric acid is made by the body from purines in food, and meats are high in purines. Some change in diet may help. Bicarbonate or citrate may be prescribed to make the urine alkaline; there is less chance for uric acid crystals to form in an alkaline urine. When necessary, allopurinol may be prescribed; the drug is often used to prevent gout attacks by reducing uric acid secretion, and it helps to reduce stone formation by the same mechanism.

Stones also may form in some people who are neither heavy calcium excreters nor uric acid excreters. And many of these people in recent trials have been helped by either allopurinol or a diuretic.

There remains another group of people who form *cystine stones*. Cystine is an amino acid constituent of protein. In a hereditary condition called *cystinuria*, the kidneys fail to normally reabsorb cystine so that its excretion in the urine is increased, and cystine stones form because of the increased urinary concentration.

The concentration can be reduced by increasing fluid intake to increase urine flow, thus providing a diluting effect. Alkalinization of the urine by regular oral intake of sodium bicarbonate also helps by making the cystine more soluble and less likely to drop out of the urine and crystallize.

Labor (See CHILDBIRTH)

Lacerations (See CUTS)

Laryngitis

The most frequent cause of laryngitis, an inflammation of the larynx, or voice box, is the common cold or other upper respiratory infection. It may also stem from excessive use of the voice, inhalation of irritating substances, and sometimes occurs in the course of flu, bronchitis, pneumonia, measles, whooping cough, diphtheria, and syphilis.

The most prominent symptom is an unnatural change of voice. Hoarseness and even complete loss of voice may occur, along with sensations of tickling and rawness and an urge to clear the throat almost constantly. In more severe cases, fever, throat pain and malaise may develop. Sometimes, if there is much fluid swelling of the larynx, there may be breathing difficulty.

WHAT TO DO: When acute laryngitis occurs in the course of a cold or other infection, it will usually disappear with disappearance of the underlying disease.

Home treatment measures include absolute rest of the voice, steam inhalation (which is soothing and often speeds recovery), and warm drinks. A cough syrup may be used to relieve cough. If a bacterial rather than viral infection is responsible for laryngitis, physician-prescribed antibiotic treatment can be effective.

Laryngotracheobronchitis, Acute (See CROUP)

Leg Cramps

Almost everyone has experienced a painful muscle cramp. When a muscle, especially one that has had relatively little use, is exercised too violently, it may react by contracting and failing to relax, producing a painful cramp.

WHAT TO DO: Heat, particularly from warm baths, is helpful, and two aspirin tablets every four hours also will be useful in relieving discomfort.

People who exercise vigorously, especially in hot weather, may develop leg cramps through loss of sodium and potassium in perspiration. The two elements are needed for efficient nervous system functioning, and with their excessive loss, faulty nerve function may overstimulate muscles, causing violent contraction and cramps. Usually, this can be avoided with well-balanced meals that include foods rich in sodium and potassium and other important substances. Such foods include chicken, eggs, liver, milk, citrus fruits, bananas, and dark-green leafy vegetables. For an attack, heat may help; so, too, stretching the muscle out as much as you can while massaging above the aching area to encourage blood flow into it.

If you tend to get leg cramps fairly often with strenuous activity, try making it a practice to do a few minutes of easy warm-up exercises beforehand and some easy cool-down exercises afterward.

Night Leg Cramps

Cramps of leg and foot muscles that awaken one from sleep constitute a common complaint. The attacks may be relatively mild and infrequent or may occur several times a night, forcing you to get out of bed, walk about, rub the muscles, and try anything to get relief.

The cause is not always clear but usually has nothing to do

with blood circulation. When poor circulation causes leg discomfort, it does so with effort rather than at rest.

WHAT TO DO: If you are taking a diuretic drug ("water pill"), that may possibly be involved because it leads to excretion of potassium, and you may benefit by increasing your intake of potassium-rich foods such as citrus fruits and bananas. Sometimes, potassium loss with a diuretic may require use of a prescribed potassium preparation.

Otherwise, many measures have been used, with varying success, to try to prevent nightly leg cramps. Some people who notice that their attacks happen more often when their feet are cool benefit by wearing socks to bed. Some benefit from elevating the legs with a pillow, which may indicate that, at least for them, pooling of blood in the legs may be a factor; the leg elevation helps return of blood from legs to heart. For some people, quinine taken at bedtime is useful.

Vitamin E has recently been reported to be effective in many cases. It is taken in the form of *d*-alpha-tocopherol acetate or succinate. Dosages used have ranged from 400 international units once a day to four times a day, although people with high blood pressure or heart problems and those with diabetes taking insulin should start with much smaller doses; and it would be wise for them to consult a physician first. Because inorganic iron combines with and inactivates vitamin E, vitamin preparations containing iron, and white bread or cereals fortified with iron, should be avoided.

Legionnaire's Disease (See PNEUMONIA)

Lice Infestation (Pediculosis)

Lice—grayish, wingless insects as small as one sixteenth of an inch in length—are parasites that live on human blood obtained by biting the skin.

Lice infestation of the scalp, common among schoolchildren regardless of socioeconomic status, is readily transmitted by personal contact and by combs, hats, and other objects. Itching is severe. If the scalp is inspected, with a lens if possible, small, ovoid, grayish-white ova (nits) can be found fixed to hair shafts, often in considerable numbers, and, unlike scales, cannot be dislodged.

Body lice infestation, which invariably produces itching, most often affects shoulders, buttocks, and abdomen. If looked for hard enough, small red marks due to bites can be found.

Pubic lice infestation usually is transmitted sexually. Itching is prominent. The lice ova are commonly attached to the skin at the base of hairs in the anogenital region. One sign of infestation may be scattered, very tiny, dark-brown specks (louse excreta) on undergarments which have come in contact with the anogenital region.

WHAT TO DO: Cure of all forms of lice infestation is rapid with a drug available on prescription. Called Kwell (1 percent gamma benzene hexachloride) it is applied once a day for two days, in shampoo, cream, or lotion form. Another application in ten days may be used to kill any surviving nits.

Because recurrence is common, it is important that possible sources of infestation such as combs, hats, clothing, and bedding be cleaned by boiling, thorough laundering and steam pressing, or dry cleaning.

"Lump in the Throat"

A sensation of having a lump in the throat, sometimes accompanied by difficulty in swallowing but with eating still possible, is one of the most common symptoms of anxiety. There is even a medical term for it: *globus hystericus*.

To be sure, there are physical diseases that can produce swallowing difficulty. In such cases, the swallowing difficulty usually begins with solid foods, progresses to liquids, causes weight loss. Most often such diseases occur in people over 40. Globus hystericus, however, tends to be more common in young adults.

WHAT TO DO: Often just recognition of the association between lump in the throat and anxiety—or in some cases an association with grief feelings—is enough to lead to its disappearance.

If it persists, or if you have any reason to believe there may be a physical cause, your physician can check, examining throat and chest. If he thinks it necessary, x-rays of the esophagus can be made or a direct examination can be performed with a flexible fiberoptic esophagoscope. If an abnormality is found, it will be treated. If not, the added reassurance that there is no physical cause can be helpful.

Lung, Collapsed (See PNEUMOTHORAX)

Measles (See CHILDHOOD DISEASES, COMMUNICABLE)

Menstrual Difficulties

Any bleeding, pain, or discharge between periods should have medical attention. Much more common problems are premenstrual tension and painful menstruation.

Premenstrual Tension

Beginning about a week to ten days before menstruation and ending within a few hours after flow begins, premenstrual tension may produce nervousness and irritability, headaches, sometimes pain in the breasts, and puffiness about the abdomen and elsewhere.

The symptoms seem to be related to fluctuations in the hormones estrogen and progesterone at this time in the menstrual cycle and to the tendency of estrogen to retain fluid in the body. Still, the exact mechanism is not known, and hormone treatment is not notably effective.

Although it is certainly discomforting, premenstrual tension does not indicate in itself any serious underlying disorder.

WHAT TO DO: If symptoms are mild, no treatment may be needed, or a mild analgesic such as aspirin, two tablets every four to six hours, can be used. For more severe symptoms, it is helpful to control the edema, or fluid retention. This can be done with a physician-prescribed diuretic ("water pill"). But often it can be accomplished more naturally, without use of a drug and possible undesirable side effects, by limiting salt intake. Salt tends to hold water in the body. And the modern American diet is loaded with salt—at least ten times more than we actually need. (In addition to its contribution to premenstrual tension, excessive salt intake is believed to be a significant cause of high blood pressure.) Any reduction in salt intake you can achieve may help considerably in relieving fluid retention and premenstrual tension symptoms. While it would be a healthy practice to put limits on salt at all times, even limitations only 24 to 36 hours before you expect symptoms can help.

Painful Menstruation

Also known as *dysmenorrhea,* painful menstruation is characterized by cramplike discomfort that may be mild to severe and is usually located in the lower abdomen or, sometimes, in the back and thighs. The pain may begin just before menstruation and persist for a few hours or through the menstrual period. Often there are other symptoms: urinary frequency, nausea, diarrhea, backache, headache, pelvic soreness.

Dysmenorrhea is *primary* when it begins at puberty; the cause is unknown. *Secondary* dysmenorrhea, which begins later in life, is usually associated with an organic cause such as pelvic inflammation, cervical stricture, abnormal position of the uterus, endometriosis (the presence of uterine tissue outside the uterus), or tumor of the uterus or ovary.

WHAT TO DO: One comforting fact about primary dysmenorrhea is that typically it ends with the first pregnancy. There is relief for it before that. In many cases, aspirin is helpful. In addition to its pain-relieving action, aspirin tends to act to counter uterine spasm and minimize clot formation. While various products are marketed as being specially designed for menstrual difficulty, you will find that commonly they contain aspirin as the main ingredient, and you will be served just as well by a less expensive form of aspirin.

Primary dysmenorrhea also may benefit from physical activity, including sports and postural exercises. For women who are sexually active and do not desire pregnancy, oral contraceptives will relieve dysmenorrhea, as they suppress ovulation, without which cramps do not occur.

For secondary dysmenorrhea, a thorough medical examination is warranted. Beyond relieving symptoms, the physician can determine and treat the underlying cause. Pelvic inflammatory disease, for example, may yield to suitable antibiotics. Endometriosis may yield to medical treatment. Other causes can be treated medically or surgically.

Migraine (See HEADACHES)

Miliaria (Prickly Heat, Heat Rash)

This itching skin eruption results from obstruction of sweat ducts and sweat retention. The trapped sweat, unable to reach the skin surface, causes at best prickling irritation and at worst severe itching.

If the duct blockage is near the skin surface, there are vesicles or blisters. Redness occurs if the blockage is deeper. The eruption may appear on the chest, back, waistline, underarms, or other areas.

Possible causative factors include skin irritation from adhesive tape, sunburn, wet compresses, diapers, exercise.

WHAT TO DO: Miliaria is a nuisance but no cause for concern. The eruption disappears within days, sometimes within hours, if the cause is eliminated.

A starch bath is often soothing. A drying lotion may provide relief. Just cool applications followed by thorough, gentle drying can help. Air conditioning is of value.

Although not often needed, your physician may prescribe a corticosteroid (cortisonelike) lotion, sometimes with added menthol.

Milk Intolerance

This is a surprisingly common problem, estimated to affect as many as 30 million Americans.

It produces abdominal bloating, unexplained cramps or diarrhea, and flatulence.

The intolerance is not allergic in nature. Instead, it involves a deficiency of an enzyme in the intestine needed to digest the lactose (sugar) constituent of milk. Without the enzyme, lactose is unabsorbed, and as it passes through the intestine causes symptoms.

The enzyme is present at birth and in childhood. But it now appears that much of the capacity to produce it is lost at an early age in many people, and victims of milk intolerance include otherwise healthy individuals who drank milk without ill effects in childhood.

TESTING FOR YOURSELF: If you have symptoms that suggest milk intolerance, a physician can make the diagnosis through a lactose tolerance test, in which you consume a specified amount of milk and measurements are then made on a sample of blood.

But you can probably establish the diagnosis for yourself. One way is to simply limit your milk intake or stop it entirely for a week and see if your symptoms disappear. Another method is to drink two glasses of cold milk (cold seems to cause more trouble than warm) on an empty stomach and your typical symptoms may appear, pointing to milk intolerance.

WHAT TO DO: Intolerance need not mean that you must steer entirely clear of milk.

Many if not most milk-intolerant people cannot handle large amounts but do well with smaller amounts in cereals and coffee, and also have less likelihood of trouble if they take the milk with meals rather than by itself. Ice-cold milk especially is to be avoided. Intolerant people, too, do well with forms of milk such as yogurt and cheese, in which part of the lactose has been converted to another substance during processing. Plans are under way for the enzyme itself to be added to commercial milk by some dairies.

You may also try an enzyme product, called Lact-Aid, now becoming available in drugstores, supermarkets, and other stores. A packet added to a quart of milk is said to supply the missing or deficient lactase enzyme in suitable quantity.

Milk Leg (See VENOUS THROMBOSIS)

Moniliasis (See VAGINAL DISCHARGE AND VAGINAL INFECTION)

Mononucleosis, Infectious

Believed to be a viral infection, infectious mononucleosis is mainly a disease of children and young adults. Its transmission is not fully understood, but when it occurs in teen-agers it is sometimes called the "kissing disease." It occurs most often in the spring of the year.

Commonly, the disease begins with malaise, fatigue, headache, and chilliness. Gland (lymph node) swellings in the neck and elsewhere are common and give the disease another name it is known by, *glandular fever.*

Mononucleosis can affect many areas of the body, producing any or many of these other symptoms: sore throat, fever, abdominal pain, nausea, jaundice, faintly red skin eruptions, eyelid swelling, severe headache, stiff neck, light sensitivity, eyeball tenderness, chest pain, breathing difficulty, and cough.

WHAT TO DO: There is no specific treatment for the disease. Bed rest, liberal fluid intake, aspirin to reduce temperature, salt-water gargles, and lozenges for sore throat may be used. If a complicating bacterial infection also should develop, an antibiotic may be needed.

The disease is usually benign, over within one to three weeks, although it may hang on longer in some cases. There is no aftermath.

Mumps (See CHILDHOOD DISEASES, COMMUNICABLE)

Muscle and Joint Pain, Tenderness, Stiffness (Fibromyositis)

Usually caused by injury, strain, exposure to damp or cold, and occasionally by infection, fibromyositis is an inflammation of muscle tissue and the connective tissue of joints and muscles.

It produces pain, often sudden in onset, which is aggravated by movement. Tenderness and stiffness also develop. Most often affected are the low back, shoulders, chest, and thighs.

WHAT TO DO: Fibromyositis may disappear spontaneously in a few days or weeks but sometimes may become chronic or reappear at intervals.

Simple home measures often can provide relief: rest, local applications of heat, gentle massage, and two aspirin or acetaminophen tablets every three or four hours.

In severe, persistent, or recurrent cases, the problem may lie with very sensitive little areas in muscles called *trigger points*. Aptly named, trigger points—like gun triggers—can fire off pain to another place, a target area.

A trigger point in the shoulder may shoot pain to neck and shoulder that may seem to be due to arthritis of the neck area of the spine—or it can cause tingling sensations in the neck and forearm, or headaches with the pain distributed to the top of the skull. A trigger point in the low back area can cause low back and sometimes sciaticalike pain shooting down the leg.

A trigger point may result from excessive exercise, a sudden twist, strain or sprain, even sleeping in poor position. Poor posture may be accountable. And fatigue, chilling, and anxiety may contribute.

Once the possibility of a trigger point is considered, you may be able to find it at home, or your physician can find it— and, in any case, if a trigger point is the problem, you will need medical help.

When a fingertip is applied firmly to a trigger point, sudden intensification of the typical pain makes the diagnosis obvious. But it may take systematic exploration to find the trigger point because it may be at a distance from the painful area.

Once the point is found, the physician can inject a small amount of a local anesthetic, such as Novocain, Xylocaine, or Carbocaine, directly into the area. Sometimes, a cortisonelike drug may be injected along with the anesthetic.

Discomfort intensifies during the injection, but pain and tenderness usually disappear within a few minutes. In some cases, a single injection may be enough; in chronic cases, a series of injections given every four to seven days may be needed for long-lasting relief.

Nail Ringworm (See RINGWORM INFECTIONS)

Nausea and Vomiting

Nausea and vomiting commonly accompany many relatively simple problems—viral infections of the intestinal tract, excessive food intake or too much alcohol, minor emotional upsets. When an infection is the cause, diarrhea often occurs.

Home treatment frequently is in order when nausea and vomiting are relatively brief, lasting no more than a day or two. If they are more persistent or accompanied by severe symptoms of another sort, medical attention is needed to determine whether there may be a problem such as an ulcer, gallbladder disease, or another digestive tract disorder. Medical attention is also called for if there is repeated nausea and vomiting after a head injury, in which case swelling of a clot between the brain and the skull may be responsible and require medical or surgical treatment. While nausea is common in the early weeks of pregnancy, if it is present after about the twelfth week, a physician should be called upon for help. It is possible in some cases for nausea and vomiting to be related to simple constipation if there has been no bowel movement for some time—but persistent vomiting, distention, and inability to move the bowel may indicate intestinal blockage.

It is also possible that a drug you may be taking—prescribed or over-the-counter—may cause nausea as a side effect. Many medications do. If this is a possibility, check with your physician. If the medication is essential, a change in dosage or a switch to another similar and equally useful drug may overcome the nausea problem.

WHAT TO DO: For home treatment of the nausea/vomiting symptom, Emetrol, available without prescription, is a useful medication, often quickly effective, acting directly on the wall of an overactive gastrointestinal tract. It appears to be free of undesirable effects.

Minimize or even avoid solid foods. With vomiting, fluids are lost, and while dehydration takes a day or more to develop, guard against it with fluids. Sip water or ginger ale. If it is difficult to keep these down, suck on ice chips. As improvement occurs, work up toward a normal diet, starting with soups, bouillon, applesauce, Jell-O, and other simple items, adding milk and milk products if they set well.

Neck Pain

Acute neck pain is a very common problem with several possible causes.

Often, it is a matter of neck muscle spasm. With such spasm

(involuntary muscular contraction), the pain is not necessarily limited to the neck. It may radiate between the shoulder blades and to the tops of the shoulders and in some cases to the upper arms. Sometimes, moving neck or shoulders may cause pain or crunching sounds in the neck muscles.

WHAT TO DO: The spasm may be set up by an injury. If it occurs in the morning, it can be due to posture during sleep and may indicate need for a firm mattress or use of a bedboard to firm your present mattress. Often replacing an ordinary pillow with a cervical (neck) contour pillow (which you may find in a medical or hospital supply house if not in regular stores) may make a marked difference.

During an acute attack, heat helps relieve both pain and spasm. Apply it as often as you find it helpful—in the form of a hot shower, hot compress, or heating pad. Aspirin or acetaminophen also helps. If you have on hand a muscle-relaxing agent such as meprobamate (Miltown, Equanil), a 400-milligram tablet four times a day during the acute attack can be useful.

Muscle spasm may sometimes set up trigger points— tender, dime-size or smaller areas—in the neck muscles which hurt and may shoot pain out when you press with your thumb on them or have someone else do so. If they are present, you may get some relief with heat. If that doesn't help enough, a physician may inject Novocain or apply a local anesthetic spray such as ethyl chloride and massage it in.

OTHER CAUSES: Flu can sometimes cause neck pain along with fever, headache, and other muscular aching. The pain will depart with the flu; meantime, a hot compress or heating pad along with aspirin or acetaminophen can help.

When neck pain results from meningitis (relatively rarely) or from arthritis of the neck which pinches a nerve (not so rare), medical help is needed.

Meningitis is likely to produce intense neck muscle spasm and stiffness, along with fever and headache, and it may be difficult to put your chin on your chest. If you have the slightest suspicion that meningitis may be involved, see a physician without delay.

When arthritis affects the neck area of the spine, nerves

emerging from the spine in that area may be pinched. The pinching can produce neck pain and may also cause pain down an arm and numbness and tingling in the arm and the hand. Tilting your head back may make you feel better—and if you place your chin and then each ear on right and left shoulders, these movements will pinch the nerves and exacerbate the symptoms if the problem is arthritis.

If nerve pinching is your problem or seems likely to be, neck x-rays will be taken to help make certain. If x-rays confirm, you may be given a more potent pain-killer and a muscle relaxant. Heat is also likely to help. In addition, you may need to wear a neck collar or, for periods at home, use neck traction with your head in a halter. The halter is attached to a system that has pulleys on a metal frame and can be hooked over a door. You can be seated. As your physician may advise, it is important that traction be applied with the neck bent downward 15 to 20 degrees or even a bit more. Your face should be oriented toward your chest with your eyes looking at something on the floor rather than straight ahead. Traction is often effective, but it should be used preferably only after x-rays show not only that the problem lies with a pinched nerve but also that no rare condition that might be aggravated by cervical traction is present.

Tension Neckache

I've left this for last but not because it is the least important kind of neck pain. On the contrary, it is common—and, in a sense, it belongs in the same category as the well-known tension headache.

As the name implies, tension headache is related to tension —emotional and muscular. So, very often, is neck pain, with or without headache. The reason lies with the *trapezius muscle*, running from the middle of the back up the shoulder tips and neck and attaching finally to the lower part of the back of the skull.

When the powerful trapezius goes into spasm, it can pull on the periosteal covering of the skull, producing a very painful constricting sensation. It is also possible for the trapezius, in spasm, to produce neck pain or pain in the upper back. And the trapezius has many opportunities for going into spasm, since commonly, when under stress, we elevate the shoulders a bit and may keep them elevated—enough to contract the trapezius long enough for it to go into spasm. The elevating action is somewhat similar to that of a cat, which, when alarmed or otherwise disturbed and getting ready to pounce or flee, arches its back and hunches its shoulders.

WHAT TO DO: Aspirin alone may not provide sufficient relief for a tension neckache. If medication alone is relied on, aspirin may have to be supplemented with a sedative or tranquilizer to help calm and relax.

But if you have no sedative or tranquilizer immediately available, you can take aspirin or acetaminophen and apply either heat or cold (whichever you find works best for you) to the muscle in the back of the neck. Massaging the back of the neck is also helpful; using your fingertips, rub the area from the back of the skull down the neck and across the top of the shoulders, repeating several times at one sitting, and repeating several times a day.

Also helpful for the acute attack and for preventive purposes as well: Take time out occasionally for just brief periods to raise your shoulders up close to your ears and then shake them down; to wiggle your shoulders and arms up and around; and to roll your head gently in circles. In these maneuvers, you contract some muscles but at the same time cause others to relax.

Neck, Stiff or Wry (Twisted)

In most cases, a stiff neck is a mild disorder. It results from a muscle cramp which can be triggered by sleeping in an abnormally cramped position, unusual exercise, a sudden twist of the neck, or a chill.

WHAT TO DO: You can usually manage this kind of neck stiffness with home measures such as hot showers, hot wet packs, and massage. Aspirin can be helpful. If the stiffness persists, it may be due to arthritis, a spinal disc, or other problem which needs medical help.

Wryneck

Wryneck, also known as *spasmodic torticollis*, is another kind of problem in which spasm or involuntary contraction of neck muscles twists the head to one side and bends the neck abnormally. Wryneck can come on suddenly or gradually. Occasionally it may be due to an infection or tumor in bone or soft tissue of the neck. Mostly, the cause is unknown. There is some opinion that emotional problems may be involved in at least some cases.

WHAT TO DO: It is sometimes possible to stop the muscle spasm at least temporarily by exerting slight pressure on the jaw on the side to which the head is being rotated.

Wryneck is not easy to eliminate completely. In some cases, injection of a local anesthetic into a tender muscle area (a trigger point) may be required.

Nosebleed (See BLEEDING FROM THE NOSE)

Nose, Foreign Object in (See FOREIGN OBJECT IN THE NOSE)

Numbness and Tingling

Almost everyone at some time or other has experienced a "pins and needles" sensation, or tingling sensation, or a brief episode of numbness in an arm or leg.

Commonly, changes in normal sensation result from accidental pressure on a nerve where it runs close to the body surface. Overindulgence in alcohol can sometimes produce areas of numbness; the numbness usually wears off by the following day. It's also possible for an unusual increase in smoking, when you are under special stress or for any other reason, to load the body with enough nicotine to interfere with circulation and produce arm or leg numbness for several hours.

Poor eating habits—perhaps during a fad diet for quick weight loss—may lead to numbness and tingling, especially when there is inadequacy of the B vitamins, and a few good balanced meals will straighten that out.

Another frequent cause is hyperventilation, or overbreathing, which is a common problem that can be responsible for many worrisome symptoms and yet, once you appreciate its role in causing numbness, tingling, or other symptoms, often can be overcome without need for medical help. (see OVER-BREATHING.)

There are other possible causes of numbness and tingling for which medical attention is usually needed:

Diabetes, undetected or uncontrolled, may be responsible.

Anemia is a cause in some cases. Because there are many possible causes for anemia, most of them simple but specific, anemia can be treated best, with quickest results, when the particular cause is determined by a blood study and specific treatment is directed at it.

Cervical syndrome: When arm or finger numbness and tingling are accompanied by one or more other symptoms such as hand or arm weakness, neck and shoulder pain, headache, and "knots" in neck muscles, the problem may be what is called the cervical syndrome, resulting from irritation of nerve roots in the cervical (neck) area of the spine. Most often, the cause of the irritation is injury, in some cases injury that may have happened well in the past. For this, treatment may include moist heat, diathermy, or ultrasound to help relieve pain and spasm; a collar to hold the neck straight for a month or more; a special cervical contour pillow to position the neck properly during sleep. If necessary, traction, special exercises, pain-killer and muscle-relaxant drugs, or injection of a local anesthetic may be used.

Polyneuritis: Numbness and tingling which may begin in

fingers or toes and extend elsewhere can be due to polyneuritis. This is a nerve inflammation that may result from injury to or pressure on nerves, or poisoning with substances such as lead, arsenic, mercury, tin, alcohol, carbon monoxide, or carbon tetrachloride. Treatment has to be directed at eliminating the cause once it is determined and may also include heat, pain-killers, and special exercises.

Raynaud's disease: Numbness of fingers and sometimes toes that is accompanied by pallor and blueness and followed by redness and throbbing pain can indicate Raynaud's disease. The disease, which involves constriction of blood vessels, is most common in young women, and its attacks may be triggered by cold or emotional disturbances and often can be relieved by warmth. Mild cases can be controlled by avoidance of cold, use of mild sedatives, and, because blood vessel constriction is involved, elimination of smoking, which has a constricting effect. A drug, reserpine, often decreases the number and severity of attacks. Recently, a simple treatment —rotating the arms in large circles—has been shown to be effective in some cases. The rotation is said to get blood to the fingers by centrifugal force.

Hypoglycemia: Numbness possibly may be due to hypoglycemia, or low blood sugar, when it occurs several hours after meals. It may then be accompanied by other symptoms. (See HYPOGLYCEMIA.)

FROSTBITE: It must be mentioned, too, that numbness with tingling sensations of toes, fingers, nose or ears, followed by burning, itching, and swelling can indicate frostbite. (See FROSTBITE.)

Osteomyelitis (See BONE PAIN)

Ovarian Cysts

A variety of cysts, or fluid-filled cavities, may develop in an ovary. Each month a cyst is formed around an egg to be released at ovulation and subsequently disappears. In some cases, for unknown reasons, such a follicular cyst may not vanish for a time, although it eventually does disappear. Occasionally, however, a follicular cyst persists, enlarges, and produces pain.

Other cysts may develop. Some may twist and, in so doing, may cause sudden severe pain in the lower abdomen, nausea, vomiting, and muscle spasm. Such cysts, which may need to be distinguished from appendicitis or intestinal obstruction by pelvic examination, require surgical removal. Some ovarian cysts can be cancerous, another reason for surgical excision.

Overbreathing (Hyperventilation)

It has been called one of the most underdiagnosed and frequently missed illnesses in medicine. Hyperventilation—breathing too deeply or too rapidly or both without conscious awareness—is capable of producing such varied symptoms as

Pounding heart
Racing pulse
Feelings of giddiness
   or light-headedness
Numbness or "pins and
   needles" sensations
Abdominal cramps
Weakness
Fainting
Chest pain similar to
   that of heart disease

Shortness of breath
Blackouts
Tension and anxiety
Swallowing difficulty
Sensation of lump in
   the throat
Muscle pains
Tremor

If you experience any of these symptoms, it is often possible for you to quickly establish whether overbreathing is the source of trouble—and, if it is, you can quickly learn how to stop attacks and even prevent them.

How can hyperventilation be responsible for such a diversity of symptoms?

We have a center in the brain that automatically regulates breathing, and normally it helps to assure that we maintain a nice balance between oxygen and carbon dioxide.

When we breathe too deeply and/or rapidly, we are actually blowing off an excess amount of carbon dioxide in the exhaled air. As a result, the level of carbon dioxide in the blood and in brain tissue falls, leading to abnormal alkalinity (respiratory alkalosis). As this happens, biochemical disturbances develop. Brain blood vessels become temporarily constricted, reducing flow of oxygen and nutrients to brain areas. Because of alkalosis, the hemoglobin in the blood temporarily loses some of its oxygen-carrying capacity. There then can follow any or many of the remarkably diverse symptoms associated with hyperventilation.

What causes hyperventilation? It sometimes results from fever, respiratory disease, or nervous system disorders. Occasionally it may stem from using large amounts of salicylate drugs for pain relief. But in the vast majority of cases, it is a response to stress.

How You Can Tell: Hyperventilation victims are usually unaware of overbreathing, although sometimes there may be deep, sighing breaths noticeable to others.

If, however, you have any suspicion that you may be experiencing episodes that might be related to hyperventilation, you need only deliberately overbreathe, taking deep and rapid breaths. Commonly, this will trigger your usual symptoms within a few minutes, sometimes even in 30 seconds. For relief—and confirmation of the diagnosis—merely rebreathe in a paper bag held over the mouth and nose, inhaling back the carbon dioxide being blown off.

What to Do: If hyperventilation is a problem for you, the very demonstration (as just described) that it is and the relief provided by rebreathing from a paper bag, indicating that the problem is not serious, may be enough to make you sufficiently conscious of the process of overbreathing that you rarely do it again.

A measure often effective in relieving or averting attacks is simply to breathe slowly through the nose with mouth tightly closed whenever an attack comes on, or threatens to, or you become aware of starting to hyperventilate. If this should fail to work, breath-holding or running in place briefly may help.

Note: Obviously, the symptoms that hyperventilation produces can have other causes. Hyperventilation warrants prime consideration because it is a common problem, easy to detect, and relatively simple to overcome. If any symptom is not duplicated when you deliberately overbreathe or not relieved when you use the measures suggested for overcoming hyperventilation, medical help may be needed.

Palpitation (See HEARTBEAT IRREGULARITIES)

Pancreatitis, Acute

Severe abdominal pain, either generalized over the whole abdomen or confined to the upper quadrants, often radiating to the back, can be due to pancreatitis, an inflammation of the pancreas. The pain steadily increases in intensity, reaches a peak in a few minutes or hours, remains severe and steady, then diminishes gradually over days or weeks as the inflammation subsides. Movement, and sometimes breathing, aggravate the pain. Sitting up or bending at the waist often relieves the pain. Fever of 100° to 102°F develops during the first few days, and nausea and vomiting are common.

Acute pancreatitis can sometimes resemble other acute problems, including peptic ulcer perforation, appendicitis, gallbladder inflammation, and even heart attack.

The most valuable diagnostic test is for an enzyme, amylase, in the blood. A marked rise in the level of the enzyme usually indicates pancreatitis.

WHAT TO DO: With any disease as painful as pancreatitis, it will be obvious that medical help is needed and should be obtained as soon as possible.

In acute pancreatitis, enzymes of the pancreas that ordinarily go into the duodenum to aid in digestion may be released into the pancreas itself and may digest some of the pancreatic tissue and blood vessels. Therefore, in treatment, no food is given by mouth, only by vein, and the stomach is kept empty by suction with a tube introduced through the nose. Both measures—by keeping food and acid out of the duodenum—help to inhibit pancreatic secretion. A drug such as atropine may be used to help further reduce pancreatic secretion. Pain may be relieved by meperidine. And antibiotics may be prescribed to counter the inflammation.

To prevent further attacks, a low-fat diet and small and frequent meals instead of three large ones may be helpful. Excessive use of alcohol unquestionably is a major factor in pancreatitis and must be avoided.

Gallbladder disease can be responsible for acute pancreatitis, since the gallbladder drainage duct and the duct carrying secretions from the pancreas join at one point. Infrequently, infectious diseases such as mumps, high blood-fat levels, overactivity of the parathyroid glands, injury, and drugs such as cortisonelike agents, some sulfa compounds, and some diuretics may be causes.

After an acute attack has subsided, it is usually wise to have gallbladder studies and remove the gallbladder if it is involved. Studies also can be done to determine if excessive blood-fat level or excessive parathyroid activity is responsible. The former can be treated medically; the latter, by surgery, removing some parathyroid tissue to bring activity down to normal.

Periods, Difficult (See MENSTRUAL DIFFICULTIES)

Peritonitis

This is an acute inflammation of the membrane lining the abdominal cavity and covering abdominal organs.

Peritonitis can produce severe abdominal pain, starting in

the lower abdomen and gradually extending upward to the right upper quadrant and middle of the abdomen. The pain increases in severity without relief and may be so intensified by movement that breathing is shallow. The abdomen becomes tight and rigid as a board.

The inflammation can be caused by infection or irritation from bacteria or chemicals reaching the membrane through an inflamed, burst appendix, perforated ulcer, ruptured gallbladder, perforated bladder, or ruptured spleen.

WHAT TO DO: Get medical attention without delay. Antibiotics can be used. Surgery is usually essential to repair the perforated area.

Phlebitis (See VENOUS THROMBOSIS)

Phlebothrombosis (See VENOUS THROMBOSIS)

"Pins and Needles" Sensations (See NUMBNESS AND TINGLING)

Pinworms (See WORM-INDUCED DISEASES)

Pleurisy

This is an inflammation of the *pleura*, the membrane covering the lungs and lining the inside of the chest. It can produce sharp, sticking chest pain that may be intensified by breathing and coughing or may be present only with deep breathing or coughing. Other symptoms can include fever, cough, chills, rapid shallow breathing.

Pleurisy can be brought on by influenza or a severe cold and can be a complication of pneumonia or other lung disease. Sometimes, it can appear for no discernible reason.

There are two forms, wet and dry.

The pleural membrane encasing each lung consists of two close-fitting layers with lubricating fluid between. If the fluid content remains unchanged, the pleurisy is called *dry*. If fluid increases abnormally, it is *wet* pleurisy or pleurisy with effusion.

In dry pleurisy, the two membrane layers may become swollen and congested, rubbing against each other as the lungs inflate and deflate, causing sharp, knifelike pain, which may radiate to shoulder, abdomen, or neck. The pain can sometimes seem like that of a heart attack, except that in a heart attack breathing makes no difference in the pain, whereas in pleurisy the pain is intensified by breathing movements of the chest.

In wet pleurisy, which often follows upon dry pleurisy, tissue fluid gets between the membranes. There may be less pain, but the excess fluid may compress the lungs and interfere with breathing, making it shallow and rapid.

If the excess fluid becomes infected and pus forms, the condition is called *empyema* or *purulent pleurisy*. Empyema produces sharp chest pain, cough, chills, fever, sweating, intense malaise, foul breath, and appetite loss.

WHAT TO DO: Prompt medical attention is needed.

Bed rest is essential. Pain can be relieved by aspirin or, when necessary, by other analgesics. Nonadhesive elastic bandages may be wrapped around the entire chest to relieve pain by limiting expansion of the chest. Coughing to drain the air passages is important and can be facilitated if the patient or someone else holds a pillow against the painful chest wall during the coughing.

When there is great difficulty in breathing caused by excessive fluid between the membranes, the removal of the fluid with a needle by a physician can produce dramatic relief. The procedure is performed with local anesthesia.

Antibiotic treatment may be used when indicated. Any underlying disease also will be treated. If there is no stubborn underlying disease, the outlook for complete recovery is excellent.

Pneumonia

Pneumonia, an infection of the lungs, can be caused by various bacteria and viruses and by oily material and other foreign matter that get into the lungs.

Bacterial Pneumonia

This is the most common type. It is infectious and can be spread from person to person, usually through the air.

The lungs are divided into five lobes. If one or more lobes are affected, the infection is called *lobar pneumonia;* infection of both lungs is called *double* or *bilateral pneumonia. Bronchopneumonia* refers to pneumonia that is localized mainly in or around the bronchial tubes; it is usually but not always milder than lobar pneumonia.

Pneumonia often begins as, or may be preceded by, a respiratory infection such as the common cold. When the lungs become involved, the disease is not difficult to identify.

There may be a sudden, shaking chill. High fever follows. Other cardinal symptoms include sharp chest pains, cough, and blood-streaked or rusty brown sputum.

WHAT TO DO: Anyone with these symptoms should get into bed and remain there, and a physician should be called immediately.

Pneumonia is an emergency disease. Although there has been some tendency since the advent of antibiotics to dismiss the disease as no longer important, it is potentially dangerous and requires prompt and adequate treatment.

A suitable antibiotic must be started at once, even while a phlegm or smear sample is sent to a laboratory. Once the particular bacterium is identified by the laboratory, the physician may change to a still better antibiotic for that organism.

Complete bed rest is required. The patient should be isolated, with few or no visitors, and masks should be worn if possible.

Plenty of liquids should be taken, and a suitable diet will be ordered by the physician. A tight chest binder against which the patient can cough may be helpful.

The outlook for pneumonia when antibiotic treatment is instituted promptly is excellent. Chances for recovery are about 95 out of 100.

PREVENTION: Good general health is an important protective factor; when the body is weakened, resistance to pneumonia organisms is lowered.

New vaccines against pneumonia are being developed. One, for example, now available to immunize against pneumococcal pneumonia, which is the most common bacterial form, is 90 percent effective and may be especially valuable for people in older age groups and those with chronic diseases such as diabetes and heart, liver and kidney disease, who may be particularly susceptible.

Legionnaire's Disease

In the summer of 1976, a mysterious epidemic of severe pneumonialike disease struck 180 persons in Philadelphia, most of whom were attending an American Legion convention. There were 29 fatalities.

The disease was characterized by fever, cough, and chest x-ray evidence of pneumonia. It took intensive investigation before a particular organism—a Gram-negative bacterium—could be not only isolated from lung tissue of disease victims but also established as the causative agent.

Much remains to be learned about the disease. Since the Philadelphia outbreak, other cases have been reported. What the prevalence may be throughout the country is not yet known.

Recently, too, researchers have been finding that there are at least two separate forms of Legionnaire's disease. Although both are caused by the same bacterium, a second form is not potentially fatal. It is more influenzalike, with the victim experiencing headache, fever, and muscle ache.

Meanwhile, progress has been made in identifying and treating the disease, including the potentially fatal form.

Tests to confirm the presence of the disease, originally developed by the National Center for Disease Control in Atlanta, now can be carried out by almost all state laboratories and many private laboratories. Other tests also are being developed.

The tests are vital. Legionnaire's disease does not respond to all antibiotics. Penicillin, for example, seems useless. Good results, however, have been achieved with certain other antibiotics—erythromycin, in particular. There have also been reports of improvement with the antibiotics chloramphenicol and tetracycline.

WHAT TO DO: Any pneumonia that produces severe symptoms is, as already noted, an emergency disease.

Along with fever, breathing difficulty, cough, and blood in the sputum, Legionnaire's disease may produce other symptoms which do not necessarily distinguish it from other forms of pneumonia: muscle pains, severe headache, vomiting, diarrhea, delirium.

Get into bed; get a physician. Antibiotic treatment may be started immediately, and the particular antibiotic may be changed according to what laboratory tests indicate.

Like other pneumonias, so with Legionnaire's disease: chances for successful recovery are greatly improved by prompt and suitable care.

Atypical (Viral) Penumonia

This type of pneumonia differs somewhat from bacterial pneumonias. Although it is often called viral or virus pneumonia, it may be caused more often by organisms called *Mycoplasma*, which are a kind of bacteria, rather than by viruses.

The onset is gradual. There are mild cases in which symptoms are much like those of the common cold. In other cases, there may be mild chills and fever. Cough is common. Sputum usually contains pus and occasionally may be bloody. Severe headache, muscle aches, and loss of appetite may be present.

WHAT TO DO: A physician should be called. Atypical pneumonia, if caused by *Mycoplasma* bacteria, usually responds well to the antibiotic tetracycline.

Even without specific medication, the disease tends to be self-limiting. Bed rest is important. Codeine or another agent may be needed for cough. Steam inhalation is useful.

Rest for a few days after fever is gone may help to avoid extended fatigue and weakness.

Aspiration Pneumonia

Aspiration, medically, means the act of breathing or drawing in. An aspiration pneumonia is one caused by foreign matter drawn into the lungs.

Aspiration pneumonia may follow anesthesia, alcoholic intoxication, convulsive disorders, and disturbances of consciousness associated with vomiting which may permit some of the vomitus to be drawn into the lungs. It may sometimes follow the improper administration of oily nose drops, especially in children and older people. Oily nose drops should be administered carefully, with the patient on his back, head tilted far back and turned to the side.

If enough foreign material reaches the lungs, infection can occur. Symptoms may include fever, chest pains, cough, and shortness of breath.

WHAT TO DO: Prompt medical help is needed. A tube may be used to remove as much as possible of the foreign material. Oxygen may be administered. If acid stomach contents have gotten into the lungs, a cortisonelike drug may be administered by injection. A suitable antibiotic can be used.

In a recent medical report, a nurse noted using the Heimlich maneuver to expel vomitus that has been aspirated into the lungs of a patient.

Pneumothorax (Collapsed Lung)

In pneumothorax (see also under CHEST PAIN, p. 34), air gets within the chest and can prevent a lung from expanding normally. With lung capacity diminished, the body does not get enough oxygen and the skin and lips turn blue (cyanosis).

WHAT TO DO: With pneumothorax, it may hurt to breathe

and the victim, already short of breath from the collapsed lung, may breathe only shallowly and even may try to hold his breath because of the pain. But that may make matters worse, creating a sense of suffocation and leading to anxiety and restlessness.

Try to relieve the pain of breathing as quickly as possible with aspirin or, preferably, something stronger such as codeine if you have any on hand. Give only very small amounts of pain-relieving medication, however; large doses can depress breathing further.

If you suspect pneumothorax, medical help is needed. The physician may administer oxygen to help relieve breathlessness and restlessness as efforts are made to determine the seriousness of the lung collapse. If small amounts of air are in the chest, they may be allowed to absorb while the patient is carefully watched.

When a large amount of air is present or continues to form, it can cause increasing pressure which further collapses the lung and even pushes the heart and other structures toward the opposite side of the chest. This is called *tension pneumothorax* and is so serious that the physician may have to use a needle and syringe to withdraw air and allow the lung to expand.

In an extreme situation, when medical help is not available at all or will not be soon enough and the patient is gasping for air and getting rapidly worse, it may be lifesaving, if you have a needle and syringe available, to insert the hypodermic needle into the side of the chest, just above a rib about four inches below the armpit on the painful side. If air hisses out, you are on target. *But this is nothing to try unless the patient is very clearly in distress and getting worse and you are absolutely certain of the cause.*

In the most serious instances of pneumothorax, a physician will insert a plastic tube into the chest under local anesthesia. To this he will attach an instrument, called the Heimlich Chest Drain Valve, which allows air to leave the chest and prevents reentry. With the valve, patients may be sent home without need for hospitalization.

Occasionally, after pneumothorax, the lung does not expand fully and surgery is necessary.

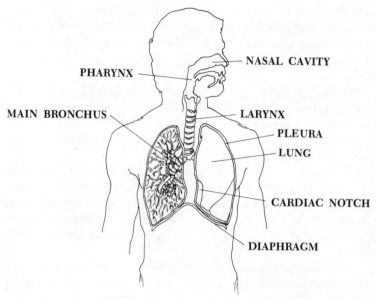

PHARYNX

NASAL CAVITY

MAIN BRONCHUS

LARYNX

PLEURA

LUNG

CARDIAC NOTCH

DIAPHRAGM

Fig. 26. Normal lungs.

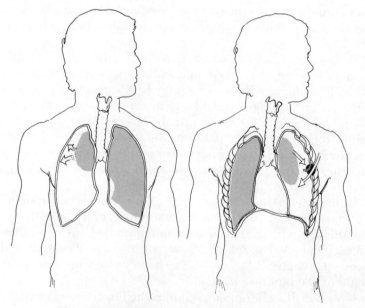

Fig. 27. Collapsed lung (pneumothorax).

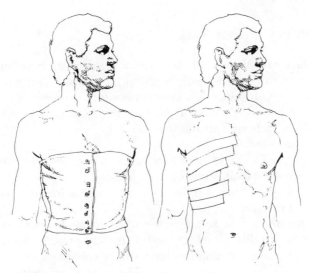

Fig. 28. Dressing for collapsed lung due to open "sucking" chest wound.

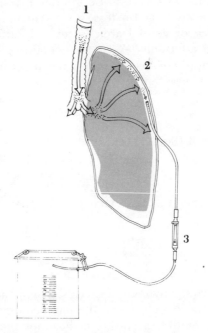

Fig. 29. Use of Heimlich valve.

Poison Ivy, Poison Oak

Contact with these and other *Rhus* (sumac family) plants at any season can produce an allergic skin reaction. The reaction may also develop through indirect contact via pets, contaminated clothing, or smoke from burning plants. It produces, after 12 to 48 hours, an itching rash which may persist for as long as two weeks.

WHAT TO DO: The irritating substance is the oily sap in leaves, flowers, fruit, stem, bark, and roots. Prompt washing of the skin with yellow laundry soap after exposure often helps prevent a reaction.

When only a few small blisters are present, warm water compresses applied for brief intervals may provide some relief. Alternatively, calamine lotion or a compress soaked in dilute Burow's solution (1 pint to 15 pints of cool water) may be applied.

If itching is too severe to be tolerated despite home measures, if there are large blisters, severe inflammation, or fever, or if the face or genital area is severely affected, seeing a physician is advisable. A cream containing a cortisonelike agent to be applied several times a day or a cortisonelike drug to be taken by mouth may be prescribed.

Prickly Heat (See MILIARIA)

Prostatitis (See URINARY TRACT INFECTIONS)

Rashes

Rashes accompany many diseases, usually along with other symptoms. These are some of the more common rash-producing illnesses, with the types of rashes they produce and other accompanying symptoms:

Measles: Pink spots, each about one-fourth inch in diameter, often start at the hairline and behind the ears and spread downward to cover the body in about 36 hours, with the spots separate at first but some, later, running together to give a blotchy look, fading after three or four days; with running nose, cough, slight fever, pains in head and back, reddened eyes. (See CHILDHOOD DISEASES, COMMUNICABLE.)

German measles: The rash is much like that of measles but the spots do not usually coalesce; they fade after two or three days; with slight cold, sore throat. (See CHILDHOOD DISEASES, COMMUNICABLE.)

Roseola: A pinkish rash appears after three or four days of fever, usually just as the fever is beginning to decline, and lasts a few days. (See CHILDHOOD DISEASES, COMMUNICABLE.)

Chickenpox: Small red spots appear on the back and chest and enlarge within a few hours, with a fluid-filled blister appearing in the center of each spot; fluid turns yellow after a day or two, a crust or scab forms and peels off in 5 to 20 days; severe itching is common. (See CHILDHOOD DISEASES, COMMUNICABLE.)

Scarlet fever: A bright red rash occurs, then fades within a week; sometimes, with it, there may be only mild fever, sore throat, swelling of neck lymph nodes; sometimes, fever may go to 105°F and there may be chills, headache, nausea, vomiting. (See CHILDHOOD DISEASES, COMMUNICABLE.)

Infectious mononucleosis: Faintly red eruptions occur with any or many other symptoms: malaise, fatigue, headache, fever, chilliness, sore throat, lymph node swelling, severe weakness, occasionally abdominal pain, nausea, jaundice, eyelid swelling. (See MONONUCLEOSIS, INFECTIOUS.)

Rocky Mountain spotted fever: Red spots, small at first and becoming larger, appear first on the extremities and spread to the trunk; other symptoms include chills, fever, headache, pain behind the eyes, joint and muscle pain, light intolerance, nausea, vomiting, sore throat, abdominal pain. (See ROCKY MOUNTAIN SPOTTED FEVER AND OTHER RICKETTSIAL DISEASES.)

Herpes zoster (shingles): Crops of blisters appear along the course of an inflamed nerve, most often in the chest, often preceded for three or four days by chills, fever, malaise, gastrointestinal disturbances. (See SHINGLES.)

Rectal Bleeding (See BLEEDING)

Rhinitis, Allergic (See ALLERGIES)

Rickettsialpox (See ROCKY MOUNTAIN SPOTTED FEVER AND OTHER RICKETTSIAL DISEASES)

Ringworm Infections

Caused by different varieties of related fungi, ringworm may affect the scalp, body, genital area, nails, and between-toes areas. (See also ATHLETE'S FOOT.)

A ringworm infection produces reddish patches, often scaly or blistered, sometimes becoming ring-shaped as the infection spreads outward. Other manifestations are itching and soreness.

The fungi are highly contagious, spread by humans, animals, combs, towels, and other objects handled by the infected.

Ringworm of the scalp, which mainly affects children, may have various manifestations, depending upon the particular fungi involved. In some cases, there may be small, scaly, semibald grayish patches with broken, lusterless hairs; in other cases, considerable shedding of infected hairs may occur.

Ringworm of the nails may lead to thickening of the nails and loss of luster. The nail plate may become separated, and the nail may be destroyed.

Ringworm of the genital area, a male problem sometimes

called "jock itch," typically affects the pubic area, may extend to the upper inner thigh and may affect both sides, but does not usually involve penis or scrotum.

WHAT TO DO: Ringworm of the scalp and nails requires medical help. Usually, it is necessary for an antifungal drug such as griseofulvin to be taken by mouth, and this has to be prescribed. For a child with scalp ringworm, sometimes a single large dose of 3 grams of griseofulvin given with ice cream or milk can be curative; if not, daily treatment can be used. For nail ringworm, persistent treatment with griseofulvin is needed, and complete eradication may require six months or even longer.

Other forms of ringworm may yield to home treatment.

An antifungal agent, Tinactin (tolnaftate), is available without prescription in cream, solution, and powder form. For "jock itch," the powder form may be best; for other infections, either the cream or the solution can be applied two or three times a day in only small amounts. Although it may take several weeks before there is complete clearance, some improvement should become apparent within a week if the treatment is working. If there is no improvement, your physician should be seen so he can prescribe other measures that will lead to eradication of the infection. Those measures may include use of griseofulvin or new and often effective locally applied medications such as miconazole cream and clotrimazole cream or lotion.

For "jock itch," tap-water compresses may be soothing until the infection clears. After bathing, it is important to gently and completely dry the area and to apply powder. Because friction and retained moisture exacerbate the infection, it is best to forgo briefs in favor of the boxer type of shorts.

Rocky Mountain Spotted Fever and Other Rickettsial Diseases

Bug-borne microscopic parasites called *rickettsiae* cause Rocky Mountain spotted fever and several other diseases.

The strain causing Rocky Mountain spotted fever is transmitted from rodent to man by the wood tick, and the principal areas for the disease are eastern and northwestern United States.

Other rickettsial diseases are *epidemic typhus*, found worldwide and transmitted by the body louse; *scrub typhus*, found mainly in the Asiatic-Pacific area and transmitted by chiggers from field mice and rats; *trench fever*, which occurs in central Europe, Africa, and North America, transmitted by the body louse; *South American spotted fever*, found in Brazil and transmitted by the rat flea; *Q fever*, found worldwide, transmitted by the wood and cattle tick; *rickettsialpox*, found in North America and Europe, transmitted by mites from house mice; and still others found in areas outside North America.

After the bite of an infected bug, a three- to ten-day incubation period follows before major symptoms of a rickettsial disease occur, although there may be loss of appetite and feelings of vague illness during the incubation period.

Onset of disease is marked by chills or chilly sensations, fever, headache, pain behind the eyes, joint and muscle pain, intolerance of light, nausea, vomiting, sore throat, and abdominal pain. Usually, about three to five days after symptoms develop, a rash appears on the wrists and ankles, and spread to the trunk and limbs, occasionally to the face.

The appearance of small red spots that become larger sores distinguishes Rocky Mountain spotted fever from the other rickettsial diseases it resembles. In trench fever, the fever first may run for three to five days, disappear for 12 to 24 hours, then recur for another three to five days. In scrub typhus and rickettsialpox, a small oval or round ulcer with surrounding redness and covered by a black scab appears at the site of attachment of the chigger or mite.

WHAT TO DO: At any suspicion of a rickettsial disease, see a physician. All of the diseases respond well to antibiotics, particularly tetracycline and chloramphenicol. If untreated, they can be serious, sometimes even fatal.

Roseola (See CHILDHOOD DISEASES, COMMUNICABLE)

Roundworm (See WORM-INDUCED DISEASES)

Scabies ("the Itch")

Now reported to have reached epidemic proportions in the United States, scabies is a skin infection caused by a parasitic mite known as *Sarcoptes scabiei*. The infection produces intense itching, which usually gets worse at night. The mite is transmitted readily, often through a whole family, by skin-to-skin contact with an infected person. Some studies indicate that up to one sixth of scabies cases result from dancing or holding hands with someone infected and even a quick handshake can transmit the infection.

Once recognized, scabies can be cured readily.

The disease originates when a female mite parasite burrows under the surface of the skin to lay eggs, leaving a sometimes-visible wavy line and, occasionally, too, a little blister or pimple at the point of entrance. During her four- to five-week life cycle, the mite lays one or two eggs a day which, after three to five days, hatch into larvae. From five days to about two weeks later, the young develop into adults, mate, and the females dig new burrows.

The main complaint is the intense itching, usually worse at night after the bed has been warmed by body heat. Wheals (hives) may develop over the entire body, regardless of where the mites are located, as a result of what is thought to be an allergic reaction to the parasites or their excretions.

Any part of the body is subject to attack, but the mites generally prefer the skin between the fingers, at the bend of the knee or elbow, on the breast and shoulder blade and, in adults, the genitalia.

If the scabies is present for several weeks, especially in a child, there may be secondary infections such as boils, impetigo, or infections of tissues around the nails. In very severe cases in both children and adults, fever, headache, and malaise may appear.

WHAT TO DO: If there is intense itching, characteristically worse at night, suspect scabies. You may or may not be able to see the telltale burrows—slightly elevated, grayish-white lines up to about a third of an inch long. Whether or not you see them, ask your physician to check for them, using a hand lens. After the disease has been present for some weeks, it may be difficult to find the burrows, since they may be obscured by scratching or other infection. Microscopic identification of the mites, however, may be made in a scraping of skin. If there is still any doubt, a trial treatment with medication known to cure the disease can be used.

The treatment is relatively simple. After scrubbing and bathing, you apply a cream or lotion containing gamma benzene hexachloride (Kwell) over the entire body below the chin. This is left on for 24 hours, then washed thoroughly. Often, this is all that is needed. When necessary, a second application can be used.

Itching sometimes may take a week or two to subside entirely. During that time, if necessary, your physician may prescribe a corticosteroid ointment for use two to four times a day.

Sometimes, any superimposed bacterial infections may need treatment with antibiotics taken by mouth, but often they clear on their own once the scabies is cured.

Note: It can be important that family members and others who have had contact with an infected individual be examined for possible scabies. All with scabies should be treated at the same time, or the infection will spread again.

Scalp Ringworm (See RINGWORM INFECTIONS)

Schistosomiasis (See WORM-INDUCED DISEASES)

Sciatica (See BACK PAIN WITH LEG PAIN)

Scrapes (See ABRASIONS)

Shingles (Herpes Zoster)

Caused by the virus of chickenpox, herpes zoster is an acute nerve inflammation with effects on the skin as well. It may occur at any age but is most common after 50.

The disease often begins with what may appear to be flulike symptoms—chills, fever, malaise, and gastrointestinal complaints. On about the fourth or fifth day, a line around the body at the chest or back, occasionally the neck, becomes red and a sudden crop of painful, small blisters appears. The blisters are on only one side of the body, usually from back around to the abdomen, following the path of the inflamed nerve. The blisters begin to dry and scab about the fifth day after they first appear.

One attack of shingles provides immunity. Most people recover without any aftermath, except for some scarring of the skin. But in some cases, most often in the elderly, a painful neuralgia may persist for months or years.

WHAT TO DO: There is no specific treatment for shingles. A cortisonelike drug, if prescribed early, may relieve pain in severe cases. Wet compresses are soothing. Aspirin alone or with codeine, taken every four to six hours, may relieve pain. Large doses of vitamin B_{12} have been reported to be helpful in some cases.

Sinusitis

The sinuses are cavities or air spaces in the skull which help to reduce the weight of the head and make the voice more resonant. They connect through small openings into the nasal passages, and normally their mucous linings produce a secretion which silently drains away through the nasal passages.

With a cold or other upper respiratory infection, the mucous membrane of the nose may swell and obstruct the sinus openings. Allergy may do the same. Bacteria then may multiply in one or more of the sinuses.

The area over an involved sinus is tender and may be swollen. When the *maxillary sinuses* in the cheekbones are affected—and this is the most common form of acute sinusitis—there will be pain in the area and headache. When the *frontal sinuses*, which are above the bony orbit of the eyes, are involved, there will be pain and headache in that area. When the *ethmoid sinuses*, located more deeply in the skull, are involved, there is pain behind and between the eyes, with a headache often described as "splitting."

WHAT TO DO: The chief aims of treatment are to improve drainage from the sinuses and control infection.

Steam inhalation is excellent for promoting drainage. Application of heat may help relieve pain. Topical vasoconstrictors such as phenylephrine spray (as in Neo-Synephrine) are helpful but should be used for no more than a week, since excessive use may have a rebound effect which may cause greater interference with drainage.

To combat the infection, a suitable antibiotic is valuable and usually should be used for no less than ten days.

CHRONIC SINUSITIS: The sinuses may become chronically infected, with thickening of the linings and sometimes production of pus. Common symptoms are nasal congestion, cough, postnasal drip, sometimes with headache (which is not as prominent a symptom as commonly believed).

Flare-ups of chronic sinusitis can be treated as just described for acute sinusitis.

The chronic disease is not easy to manage. Home humidification during winter months can help. If allergy is involved, the cause can be determined and eliminated, or combatted by desensitization treatment. In some cases, minor surgery to remove nasal polyps, drain the sinuses by creating new openings into them, or correct a deviated septum (the plate of bone and cartilage that divides the nasal cavity) may be needed. Sometimes cauterization of boggy turbinate structures in the nose may help to establish drainage. Infected teeth should be treated.

It's also good practice to blow the nose properly—never violently, always one nostril at a time with the mouth wide open. This may help to clear the sinus passages.

Climate is important in sinusitis, with the condition often aggravated in cold, moist areas.

Skin, Foreign Object in (See FOREIGN OBJECT IN THE SKIN)

Sleeping Problems (See INSOMNIA)

Splinter

To remove a splinter, wash your hands and the area around the splinter with soap and water. Sterilize a needle and a pair of tweezers—either by boiling for ten minutes in water or heating to redness in a gas flame, electric burner, or match flame and cleaning off the black carbon deposit with sterile gauze.

After allowing it to cool, use the needle to loosen the splinter from the skin and slide the point of the needle sideways under the splinter to elevate and remove it. If it doesn't come out, use the tweezers to aid removal. Wash the site a second time with soap and water.

If the splinter is lodged too deeply or is otherwise not readily removed, see a physician.

If the skin is already infected, do not attempt to remove the splinter. If you were to insert a needle into an infected area, you might spread the infection further and cause blood poisoning. See a physician.

If medical help is not available, treat the infection as a boil (see BOILS AND CARBUNCLES), with soaks until it drains, at which time the splinter should surface and be expelled spontaneously.

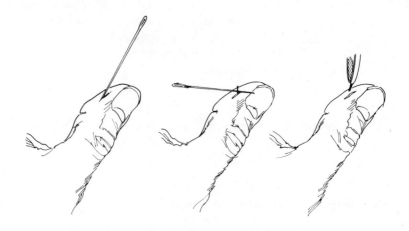

Fig. 30. Removing a splinter.

Splinting (See FRACTURES, DISLOCATIONS, SPRAINS, AND STRAINS)

Sprains and Strains (See FRACTURES, DISLOCATIONS, SPRAINS, AND STRAINS)

Stings (See INSECT AND OTHER BUG BITES AND STINGS)

Stomach Upset (See GASTRITIS, ACUTE; GASTROENTERITIS, ACUTE; INDIGESTION)

Stomatitis, Aphthous (See CANKER SORES)

Stroke

A stroke—also known as a *cerebrovascular accident (CVA)* and once called *apoplexy*—occurs either because of rupture of a brain artery, which leads to bleeding within the brain, or because of a blood clot that forms in an artery and interferes with circulation to a part of the brain.

The indications of a stroke will depend on which part of the brain is affected.

The victim's face may become very red; the eyeballs may be prominent, and the pupils of the eyes unequal in size. One side of the body may become weakened or paralyzed. Speech may be affected. The mouth may be drawn to one side. There may be difficulty in breathing or swallowing. In some cases, there may be unconsciousness.

WHAT TO DO: Call a physician or ambulance immediately.

While waiting for medical help, provide some covering, not too heavy. Loosen any tight clothing. Position the victim on his side so secretions can drain from the side of the mouth. Give no fluids by mouth unless the victim is conscious and able to swallow normally.

If the victim should stop breathing, lift up his neck with one hand and push his forehead backward and down with the other hand. This opens the airway, and breathing may start. Reach into the mouth to pull the tongue forward—it may have been swallowed.

If breathing does not start, begin rescue breathing immediately. Pinch nostrils shut with fingers of one hand and blow air into mouth. When the victim's chest moves up, take your mouth away and let the chest go down by itself. With your first four breaths, do not wait for the victim's chest to fully deflate before blowing into his mouth again.

Little Stroke

A major development in recent years has been recognition that although a major stroke may seem to develop suddenly, the stroke process is not necessarily sudden and often provides warning indications—or "little strokes."

Such warnings point to impairment of blood flow to a brain area. They take the form of brief episodes of weakness, numbness, or heaviness on one side of the body, dizziness, blurring of vision, seeing bright lights, memory disturbance, speaking or writing difficulty.

WHAT TO DO: Little strokes provide opportunity in many cases now to prevent an approaching major stroke.

Any one or a combination of the symptoms should be a signal to notify your doctor or go to a hospital. Special x-rays of neck arteries leading to the brain and of other arteries or other tests can be performed.

If the tests indicate that the cause of the symptoms is a clot in an artery of the neck or other accessible site, it may be decided to remove the clot. Or if the artery has become very much narrowed, the deposits may be reamed out or the artery section bypassed with a new channel, which may be a vein taken from elsewhere in the body or a prosthetic tube graft.

Recently, even when obstruction turns out to be located in vessels deep within the brain, it has become possible to solve the problem in many cases. In a four- to five-hour procedure called *cerebral revascularization*, using an operating microscope and other microsurgical techniques, through an opening made in the skull, a segment of a scalp artery is connected with microsutures to a segment of the middle cerebral artery, which extends over the brain. This creates a bypass of the circulation beyond an obstruction and connects two arteries that rarely become obstructed. According to reports at a recent international symposium on 400 patients so treated and followed for two and a half years on average, strokes occurred in only 3 afterward, with others experiencing great reduction of little strokes and in most cases their near elimination.

Sty

A sty is an infection of one or more of the sebaceous (oil) glands of the eyelid. It may begin, before the sty is visible, with pain in the lid, a sensation of something in the eye, or tearing. Then pain and redness of the lid margin follow, along with the appearance of what looks like a pimple.

WHAT TO DO: Often, a sty can be localized by warm compresses applied for ten minutes three or four times a day. Use a tablespoon of Epsom salt (magnesium sulfate) to a quart of water. Wet some sterile gauze with the solution and place it on the closed eye. It is most convenient to lie down while doing this. As soon as suppuration (pus formation) is shown by the appearance of a central yellow area, a physician can make a small incision and remove the contents, or the sty may open and drain by itself.

If you choose to see a physician as soon as you become aware that a sty is forming, he may be able to prevent pus development by prescribing an antibiotic ointment to be applied to the area.

Sugar, Low Blood (See HYPOGLYCEMIA)

Sunburn

In a mild case of overexposure to the sun, there are redness, itching, and mild pain. No treatment may be needed. You can, however, obtain some relief by applying cold cream, mineral oil, or talcum powder.

Any preparation containing an anesthetic should be used very cautiously if at all—and if used should be applied only once, for the anesthetic may be toxic to the skin or you may be allergic to it.

If the skin is blistered or extensively burned, you can apply a cold compress of water, whole milk, or saline solution (one teaspoon of salt to a pint of cool water).

Severe or extensive sunburn with much blistering needs prompt medical attention both for pain relief and to prevent bacterial infection.

PREVENTION: The most effective prevention lies in keeping

the length of first exposures at the beginning of summer limited to about 15 minutes, with gradual increases of 5 to 10 minutes until the skin has sufficiently thickened and tanned. Remember that sunburn can follow exposure even on a cloudy day; burning rays can penetrate clouds. Remember, too, that late mornings to midafternoons (about 10 A.M. to 4 P.M.) are periods of most intensive sunshine.

Sunburn protection preparations vary in effectiveness. Most contain oils to reduce skin tightness. Some contain effective screening agents such as PABA (para-aminobenzoic acid). Check labels before buying.

Apply an effective preparation 30 to 60 minutes before you're exposed to the sun so the protective agents have a chance to bind to the skin (a process that takes about 30 minutes). Otherwise, perspiration will wash them away.

Most people tolerate PABA well. If you do not, you can use a preparation containing a benzophenone or titanium dioxide sunscreen.

Sunstroke (See HEATSTROKE)

Suturing (See CUTS)

Swallowed Objects (See FOREIGN OBJECTS, SWALLOWED)

Swallowing Difficulties (Dysphagia)

The usual complaint is that food "gets stuck" on the way down, and the feeling may or may not be accompanied by pain.

This is a different complaint from that of a feeling of having a lump in the throat (see p. 250).

Difficulty in swallowing has many possible causes, including muscle and nervous system disorders or organic problems in the throat, the esophagus, and nearby organs.

The condition is not of such an emergency nature that it requires seeing a physician within the hour, but it does need careful medical investigation and suitable treatment. Thorough diagnostic studies are warranted, since one cause of dysphagia is cancer of the esophagus. Recently developed fiberoptic instruments have made examination of the esophagus relatively easy.

Swelling with Fluids (See EDEMA)

Syphilis (See VENEREAL DISEASES)

Tapeworm (See WORM-INDUCED DISEASES)

Tennis Elbow (See ELBOW, TENNIS)

Threadworm (See WORM-INDUCED DISEASES)

Throat, Lump in (See "LUMP IN THE THROAT")

Throat, Sore

Just like colds, most sore throats—as many as four of every five—are caused by viruses, and there are no antibiotics or specific drugs to cure them. Sore throats on occasion also can be caused by excessive smoking, coughing, or shouting.

"Strep" throat is a sore throat brought on by streptococcal bacteria, and this type requires treatment with a suitable antibiotic. If uncontrolled, it has potential for leading to rheumatic fever or kidney disease complications.

WHAT TO DO: Most sore throats can be treated at home. But a strep throat does require medical attention, as indicated.

For accurate diagnosis of a strep throat, a culture is needed. That takes 48 hours, since bacteria recovered from the patient must be grown on a laboratory plate. Your physician may do the culture in his office laboratory, or he may send you to an outside laboratory. As a time- and money-saving measure, many physicians now will have you go directly to a laboratory for a culture, avoiding an office visit, which may be needed only if the culture is positive, indicating strep throat.

Under certain conditions, it is possible for you to suspect strep throat and arrange with your physician for a culture to be taken. One such condition is the appearance of a skin rash along with the sore throat. Another is your awareness of having been exposed to strep infection. Also, if you have had rheumatic fever or kidney disease (nephritis) in the past, your physician may even start antibiotic treatment before getting culture results in order to be on the safe side.

You can also have reason to suspect the possibility of strep throat if, using a good light, you see, in the back of the throat, any pus or yellow or white mucus that may have a cobblestonelike appearance. Another possible reason for suspicion is a fever greater than 101°F, although flu can produce fevers up to 104° (along with other symptoms).

On the other hand, if your sore throat is accompanied by runny nose, headache, muscle aches and pains, cough or hoarseness, it is not likely to be a strep throat, and you will probably be safe in trying home treatment.

You can use aspirin—two tablets every four hours, if needed, for an adult; a lesser amount for a child—to relieve fever, pain, and aches. Gargle with warm salt water (a teaspoonful of salt to a glass of water) every few hours; it's a cheap treatment and safe, usually as good as lozenges, syrups and the like, although the latter have the advantage that you can take them with you. Use lozenges, etc., if they help. Rest your voice as much as possible. A vaporizer helps by keeping the throat moist. Take more fluids than usual, including frequent sips of hot liquids. Stop, or at least reduce, smoking. Keep track of your temperature, checking and recording it two or three times a day.

If temperature climbs above 101° several times a day, if throat pain is increasing not decreasing after a few days, if earache develops, or if you experience shortness of breath or chest pain, check with your physician. Check, too, if otherwise, the sore throat hangs on for more than two weeks.

Thrombophlebitis (See VENOUS THROMBOSIS)

Tingling (See NUMBNESS AND TINGLING)

Toenail, Ingrown

This problem is almost always caused by improper toenail clipping or poorly fitting shoes. It can be prevented by wearing suitable shoes and by keeping the nails short, with the sides a little longer than the middle.

WHAT TO DO: If a toenail is only slightly ingrown, you may be able to insert a tiny bit of cotton that has been soaked in castor oil under the ingrown edge of the nail. Apply a pad of clean gauze to protect the nail from pressure.

A badly ingrown toenail should always be treated by a physician or podiatrist; otherwise a serious infection may develop.

Toothache

WHAT TO DO: Try using dental floss to clean between the affected tooth and its neighbors; frequently, impacted food may be contributing to the pain. Dentists are often called about a toothache by patients who—because they have either been rushing to get ready for a trip or been extremely busy for other reasons—have been eating rapidly, chewing poorly, and not cleaning their teeth adequately. Frequently, tying a knot in a piece of dental floss and dragging it between the aching tooth and its neighbors removes a food particle which relieves the pain.

Check the mouth under a good light. If you see no cavity or swelling, apply an ice bag or cold compress against the jaw on the affected side. If this does not help, heat may. Use a hot water bottle or warm compress.

If you see a cavity, clean it out gently with sterile cotton on the end of a toothpick. Then saturate another tiny bit of sterile cotton with oil of cloves and pack it gently into the cavity with a toothpick, being careful not to let the oil of cloves touch the tongue or inside of the mouth, since it burns. If packing does not provide sufficient relief, add hot or cold applications.

Those are steps to take to get relief when a toothache strikes in the middle of the night (as it often does) or at another inconvenient time or place when you can't reach a dentist. Usually, when a toothache occurs, it means that dental care is going to be needed sooner or later—and, usually, the sooner the better.

Commonly, a toothache indicates *pulpitis*—an inflammation of the dental pulp, the soft tissue within a tooth. Pulpitis may result from thermal irritation or from an accidental injury that inflicts violence on a tooth. Grinding the teeth during sleep can irritate or inflame the pulp. A fracture of a tooth, even a hairline fracture, can expose the pulp and lead to inflammation. Most often, pulpitis results from infection and inflammation following decay.

When pulpitis is present, there may at first be only some sensitivity to cold, with pain lasting only a few minutes and then disappearing. Later, pain will appear without apparent cause, last longer, and tend to occur more often when you are lying down. There may be swelling of the face. The pain can be sharp, stabbing or throbbing, and sometimes may be difficult to pinpoint.

If not treated, the infected tooth may become abscessed and its removal may be necessary.

Pulpitis can be reversible or irreversible. In reversible pulpitis, pulp and nerve can be saved and restored to good condition. The dentist may seal off the exposed pulp after applying an antibacterial agent. When the pulpitis has advanced too far and the pulp cannot be saved, root canal work may be needed to remove the pulp and sterilize and fill the canals, leaving the tooth still alive, attached to bone, and capable of functioning for a long time.

Tooth, Knocked-Out

If your child has a permanent tooth accidentally knocked out, or if you yourself should be the victim, get to a dentist as soon as possible for the best chance of successful reimplantation, carrying the tooth with you, as to be described.

If a tooth can be reimplanted within about half an hour, there is a possibility that the interior pulp will survive. But even beyond that time, after periods of up to six hours, the outer periodontal tissue may survive and allow successful reattachment.

If there is going to be a delay, try placing the tooth in the socket yourself. If that does not work, place the tooth in a container of water or wrap it in a cloth wetted well with water to which a little salt has been added, and get to the dentist. Keeping a knocked-out tooth moist is an important factor for successful reimplantation.

Traveler's Diarrhea (See DIARRHEA)

Trench Fever (See ROCKY MOUNTAIN SPOTTED FEVER AND OTHER RICKETTSIAL DISEASES)

Trichinosis (See WORM-INDUCED DISEASES)

Trichomoniasis (See VAGINAL DISCHARGE AND VAGINAL INFECTION)

Turista (See DIARRHEA)

Typhus (See ROCKY MOUNTAIN SPOTTED FEVER AND OTHER RICKETTSIAL DISEASES)

Ulcer

Your chances of getting a peptic ulcer at some time in your life are about 1 in 10. And whereas, until recently, only 1 in 20 ulcer patients was a woman, today nearly 1 in 2 is.

The reason for the rising incidence in women is not known, although there are theories that it may be due to increasing use by women of cigarettes and alcohol, which may irritate the stomach lining.

It is also being recognized more and more that ulcer in children is not as rare as has been believed, and many a child's chronic stomachache may be a symptom of an ulcer.

A *peptic ulcer* (*peptic* = due to stomach juices; *ulcer* = an erosion) may range in size from a just discernible sore to a crater an inch or more wide and half an inch deep. If it occurs in the stomach, it is called a *gastric* or *stomach ulcer*. Far more commonly, it develops in the duodenum, the part of the small intestine closest to the stomach, which makes it a *duodenal ulcer*.

Ulcers most often develop between the ages of 25 and 40, although they may appear much earlier or much later. The peak age for children is 7 to 9.

The typical symptom is pain in the upper abdomen, which

comes on one to four hours after eating and is relieved by food or antacids. Burning or gnawing in character, the pain comes and goes for about half an hour, often appearing in the middle of the night. Commonly, for some weeks before the typical pain appears, there may be frequent episodes of heartburn and belching. There may also be general abdominal discomfort, diarrhea, nausea, and vomiting.

An ulcer can be demonstrated by x-ray and fluoroscopic studies after a swallow of barium. The ulcer can actually be seen directly and even photographed through a flexible fiberoptic gastroscope, which is easily passed through the mouth into the stomach and duodenum.

What causes a peptic ulcer?

The stomach produces hydrochloric acid and digestive enzymes to aid digestion. Even when the stomach is empty, there is a normal, intermittent flow which becomes much greater with a meal.

The acid, strong enough to dissolve even iron, does not dissolve the stomach itself because of the protective effect of the mucus secreted by the stomach's mucous glands. There is also mucous protection in the duodenum; and in addition, bile from the liver and gallbladder is alkaline and neutralizes the acid.

An ulcer may develop if there is an excess secretion of acid by the stomach or an alteration of the mucous coating.

Some ulcer patients have been found to have two to four times as many acid-secreting cells as normal. The large number, it is believed, could be the result of hereditary influences. Or extra cell formation may occur because nerve impulses through the *vagus nerve* are excessive, calling for increased acid secretion, which may trigger development of more cells as well as greater secretion from existing cells.

The vagus nerve overactivity leading to excessive acid secretion sometimes may be the result of disease elsewhere, such as diabetes or chronic lung disease, which stimulates the nerve. Acid production also may be increased by alcohol, smoking, nervousness, tension, rage, or fear.

The *mucosa*, or stomach-lining cells, may be affected by alcohol and by drugs such as aspirin and cortisonelike agents.

There are still many mysteries surrounding peptic ulcer. One puzzle is why ulcer symptoms peak in autumn and spring and bleeding from an ulcer is most frequent between September and January.

WHAT TO DO: The suspicion of an ulcer calls for medical examination, and if an ulcer is found, medical treatment is needed.

The basic principles of treatment include rest, both physical and mental, and reduction of excessive acid secretion in order to allow healing.

For *gastric ulcer,* two to three weeks of bed rest may be needed, sometimes in a hospital. Stomach ulcers need close checking. It used to be thought that they led to stomach cancer, which is not true. But what looks like stomach ulcer may sometimes be a cancer that has produced an area of ulceration. So, for a gastric ulcer, after two to three weeks of bed rest and treatment, the ulcer may be checked again by x-ray or gastroscopy. If healing or marked improvement has not occurred by then, malignancy may have to be considered and surgery may possibly be needed.

For *duodenal ulcer,* although hospitalization for a week or two may sometimes be desirable, especially if there is much pain, often acute symptoms can be brought under control by seven to ten days of rest at home, eating a reasonable diet.

Although special bland diets were once considered essential, there is no evidence that they are particularly helpful, and there is now a tendency to allow an ulcer patient to eat whatever he likes and agrees with him, within reason.

Many physicians recommend eating frequent small meals rather than three large ones so there is usually food in the stomach to absorb the acid. Usually, an ulcer patient will be told to avoid coffee (both regular and decaffeinated, since both have been found to stimulate acid production), tea, cola and cocoa, and to drink alcoholic beverages, if at all, with food and in moderation.

Treatment is also likely to include antacids to relieve symptoms (there is some evidence that they help promote ulcer healing as well). An antacid often used is a combination of aluminum hydroxide and magnesium trisilicate, which is less likely to cause constipation than is aluminum hydroxide alone. A liquid antacid is usually more effective than tablets, even if not as convenient.

Other drugs may be prescribed, including anticholinergics to delay stomach emptying and antispasmodics to relax stomach and intestinal muscles. Sedatives may sometimes be used to allay anxiety and tension. Also in increasing use is a newer medication, called cimetidine, which partly blocks release of stomach acid.

COMPLICATIONS: Although far from inevitable, complications sometimes develop.

Perforation is one. The ulcer penetrates through the stomach or duodenal wall so secretions and contents spill into the abdominal cavity. There is usually agonizing abdominal pain. Commonly, breathing becomes shallow, beads of sweat appear on the forehead, and the entire abdomen becomes boardlike. Later, peritonitis—inflammation of the membrane lining the abdomen—may develop. Perforation requires immediate surgery for repair of the penetration.

Hemorrhage is another complication. The bleeding develops when a nearby blood vessel is eroded, its wall eaten away. There may be no pain felt when bleeding occurs. The bleeding may manifest itself through the vomiting of blood or darkbrown (like coffee grounds) stomach contents or the passage of black, tarry stools. In some cases, the bleeding may not show itself, and the only symptoms may be weakness, dizziness, sometimes fainting. Medical measures, including blood or plasma transfusions or intravenous infusions of dextrose and saline, and liquid feedings, may control the bleeding. If not, surgery may be needed.

Still another complication is *obstruction*. An ulcer sometimes may cause spasm, scarring, or inflammatory swelling at the outlet of the stomach or in the duodenum, resulting in partial or complete blockage. Symptoms may include vomiting of food from previous meals and foul, gaseous belching. Medical measures often can relieve obstruction at least partially within 96 hours and entirely after about a week. But when obstruction cannot be so relieved, surgery is needed.

Unconsciousness

Loss of consciousness has many possible causes, ranging from skull fractures, stroke, diabetic coma, intoxication, and poisoning to fainting.

WHAT TO DO: If you see someone eating and fall unconscious, or if you find someone unconscious in or near a dining area, and breathing is absent, 98 percent of the time the problem is choking. Apply the Heimlich maneuver (p. 44).

In other situations, look at the lips: if they are blue, check breathing and pulse. Apply artificial breathing (p. 49) or, if necessary, because there is neither breathing nor pulse, use CPR (cardiopulmonary resuscitation) (p. 52).

Have an ambulance called.

Make the victim as comfortable as possible. If vomiting occurs, turn his head to one side to prevent choking, and clear the mouth of vomitus. Loosen any tight clothing.

Unless absolutely necessary, do not move the victim, because of the possibility he may have a skull fracture or other serious injury.

Do *not* give whiskey or water to an unconscious person.

Look for clues that could be helpful for the physician, rescue squad, or emergency room. Smell the victim's breath for a strong odor of alcohol, but do not readily pass off the problem as alcoholism; that may be a red herring. The odor of acetone (major ingredient of fingernail polish remover) could indicate diabetic coma (very high blood sugar level). A red face, very dry skin, and erratic breathing can also point to diabetic coma.

Carefully check the head and scalp for a cut or bruise indicating head injury. Treat any bleeding (see BLEEDING). If possible, check the arms for scars or black and blue marks that might indicate a drug habit.

Look for any ID bracelet or medical card or other indication that the victim is diabetic, epileptic, or has another illness.

Urethritis (See VENEREAL DISEASES)

Urinary Tract Infections

Urinary tract infection, almost always in the bladder or the kidneys, is the most common bacterial infection affecting the human body. It is about ten times more frequent in women and girls than in men and boys, largely because of anatomical difference.

In both sexes, urine is produced in the two kidneys, located in the back—in the flanks slightly beneath the lower ribs. Flowing from the kidneys through two long narrow tubes, called *ureters*, urine enters the bladder, low in the midline of the abdomen, where it is stored. For urination, valves open and the bladder drains, with urine flowing to the outside through a tube, the *urethra*.

In women, the urethra is short and straight and empties near the front of the vagina. In men, the urethra is much longer and curved, passing through the penis, and it is relatively difficult for bacteria to enter the bladder. In women, however, it is much easier for bacteria to move up from the skin in the vaginal region, which cannot be kept sterile, through the short, straight urethra to the bladder.

Infections are frequent during pregnancy, possibly because the expanding uterus may press on the ureters, interfering with normal urine flow. Any such interference—from this cause or from others such as compression by uterine tumors or blockage caused by a stone—may encourage bacterial multiplication in the more or less stagnant urine.

Another frequent problem for women is the bladder infection known as *honeymoon cystitis*. Infection may develop after intercourse as manipulation and irritation in the vaginal area foster bacterial penetration up the urethra to the bladder.

SYMPTOMS: In either sex, the symptoms of acute urinary tract infection are difficult to ignore.

In acute bladder infection (*cystitis*), there is usually burning on urination or painful urination with urgency and frequency. Often there is *nocturia* (excessive urination at night). Low back pain is frequent. Blood may also appear in the urine, particularly in women.

Usually with acute kidney infection, there are other symptoms as well: chills, fever, high back pain or loin pain on either side, nausea and vomiting.

WHAT TO DO: For some relief of symptoms until you can see a physician, you can take aspirin for pain and sitz baths for burning. Increase your liquid intake in order to help wash out the urinary tract—but avoid alcohol, tea, and coffee during the illness, since they tend to irritate the urinary tract. Rest in bed if there is fever.

You will want to get medical attention as soon as possible, since a physician can prescribe both curative and more potent symptom-relieving measures.

For cure, an antibacterial agent—a sulfa drug or an antibiotic—is used and may bring relief of symptoms as well as begin to eliminate infection within 24 to 48 hours.

For symptom relief before the antibacterial drug can take hold, a variety of preparations are available. Many counter muscle spasm in the urinary tract and help to relieve urinary frequency and urgency. For pain, a topical urinary analgesic such as methylene blue or phenazopyridine may be used.

If you experience frequently recurring urinary tract infections, urologic investigation may be necessary to determine if there may be any correctable urinary tract obstructions or other abnormalities fostering the repetitions.

If you're a woman who experiences frequent bouts of cystitis, you may find it worthwhile to abstain from tub bathing in favor of showers. In at least one research study, the great majority of a group of women who had experienced multiple recurrences (as many as ten in some cases) remained free of them as long as they avoided tub baths.

If your infections could be linked to intercourse, emptying the bladder soon after coitus may help. It is much more likely to be effective, recent research indicates, if done within 15 minutes afterward rather than later.

A NOTE FOR MEN: *Prostatitis*—an inflammation of the prostate gland—sometimes produces symptoms like those of urinary tract infection, along with other symptoms as well. There may be urinary frequency, painful urination, and in some cases fever and pain in the scrotum, rectum, or the area between scrotum and rectum. Sometimes, there may be slight drainage from the penis. The symptoms can be similar to those of mild gonorrhea, but gonorrhea can be ruled out by medical examination.

Prostatitis may require antibiotic treatment. It sometimes is relieved with prostate massage. Hot baths often bring comfort.

Urticaria (See HIVES AND GIANT HIVES)

Vaginal Discharge and Vaginal Infection

Vaginal infection (*vaginitis*) is a common problem—but vaginal discharge does not necessarily mean infection. A small vaginal discharge is normally present in all women during the reproductive, menstruating years.

Cells are constantly being cast off from the cervix and vagina, leading to occasional discharge of a small amount of white or grayish, semisolid material. A watery or mucoid secretion also may normally follow sexual stimulation. About the time of ovulation, some blood may tinge the discharge. Normally, too, a discharge occurs just before a girl begins to menstruate. Pregnancy brings an increase in the discharge. Oral contraceptives commonly produce discharge.

Normal vaginal discharges are usually small in amount, whitish or clear, free of pus and, except at ovulation, free of blood. They are also unaccompanied by itching or irritation.

Abnormal discharge often is the result of infection of any of several varieties. But we should note, first, that surprisingly often it can be unintentionally self-inflicted.

For one thing, excessive use by fastidious women of vaginal deodorants, sprays, creams, jellies, or powders can sometimes lead to vaginal inflammation and discharge—and at that point there is often a tendency to use more of what is causing the trouble.

For another, a not uncommon cause of discharge is a foreign object in the vagina—a forgotten tampon, diaphragm, or pessary. Often such discharge is tinged with blood and foul-smelling.

One of the most common causes of infectious vaginal discharge is *Trichomonas*, an organism a little larger than a red blood cell. The discharge is frothy or foamy, yellow-white or greenish, and associated with itching and burning or soreness. *Trichomoniasis*, as this infection is called, commonly occurs or recurs after sexual intercourse. A man may carry the infection without being aware of it, since he is free of all symptoms.

Monilia is another very common offender. A fungus, it causes an infection known as *moniliasis* (*candidiasis* is another name) that produces a white, thick, creamy or curdlike discharge, usually without odor but with intense itching and sometimes burning or soreness. Moniliasis is more likely to occur in pregnancy and in diabetic patients than in others but also can occur in women using oral contraceptives and commonly is a side effect of antibiotic treatment.

Hemophilus vaginitis, caused by bacteria, produces a scant to profuse, watery, gray or white discharge which may have an unpleasant odor. Only rarely is there itching, and burning or soreness, if either occurs, is usually mild. Like trichomoniasis, this type of infection requires treatment of the sex partner; otherwise there can be a "ping-pong" effect with organisms passed back and forth.

Nonspecific vaginitis is also common. This infection, which produces a foul discharge, appears to be due to a mixture of bacteria.

WHAT TO DO: Although vaginal infections are not serious and do not spread elsewhere, they are of course discomforting.

Occasionally, a vaginal infection may disappear on its own. A vinegar douche—made with two tablespoonsful of vinegar to a quart of warm water—may be helpful if used once or twice a week but may increase discomfort if tissues are inflamed.

There are specific treatments a physician can prescribe, depending upon the organisms involved. If your problem persists for more than a week or two, you should get medical help. And you may do well to get it earlier to speed relief.

For trichomoniasis, a usual prescription is metronidazole taken by mouth for seven to ten days, and the same treatment is recommended for husbands. The drug should not be used during pregnancy. Instead, a local preparation can be used at that time—vaginal tablets of diiodohydroxyquin or vaginal suppositories of furazolidone.

For moniliasis, nystatin or gentian violet suppositories may be used. Another often-effective treatment is with a cream containing miconazole nitrate, which may relieve itching within three or four days.

Hemophilus vaginitis can be treated effectively with a sulfa drug in the form of a pill or a vaginal suppository, or with a penicillin compound, ampicillin.

For nonspecific vaginitis, vaginal application of a triple sulfonamide cream morning and night can be effective.

Some other matters you should know about—both for overcoming and preventing vaginal infection:

• Avoid wearing pants or body suits that fit tightly in the crotch and thighs; they may retain moisture and heat, both of which encourage organism growth.

• When taking a prescribed treatment for vaginal infection, take it for the full prescribed time. If you stop short when symptoms are relieved, the infection may not have been wiped out completely and may flare again.

• It's a good idea to eat yogurt several times a day whenever you have to take an antibiotic for an infection anywhere in the body, especially if you have had trouble with moniliasis before. If you can't tolerate yogurt, your physician can suggest tablets that help to replace the good normal bacteria in the vagina that may be wiped out as an antibiotic, while doing its job of fighting infectious organisms, cuts a swath through the beneficial as well.

Special note: A vaginal discharge may be associated with gonorrhea (see next section). If there is any possibility of this, don't delay seeking medical help.

Venereal Diseases

What is most dangerous about a venereal disease is ignoring it. Recognized and treated early, venereal diseases can be rendered harmless.

All such diseases require medical treatment.

Gonorrhea

Long the most common venereal disease, gonorrhea ("clap") is caused by the bacterium *Neisseria gonorrhoeae* and is acquired by physical contact with someone who has the infection.

In men, symptoms commonly start with some pain and burning on urination, from two days to two weeks (most often, within five days) after contracting the infection. A thick mucous discharge from the penis is present. If treatment is delayed, there may be increasing difficulty in urinating, which may be due to spread of the infection to the prostate. Also, fever, pain, and swelling and tenderness of the testes and scrotum may develop.

In women, symptoms are less obvious and in some cases there are no symptoms at all. When symptoms occur, they are often mild to begin with: slight burning on urination, vaginal discharge, and later, in some women, lower abdominal pain. If not treated, gonorrhea can lead to severe inflammation of all pelvic organs, with possible abscess formation, scarring, and sterility.

For certain diagnosis, a physician will need to obtain a specimen of discharge from the penis or from inside the vagina. A suitable antibiotic in adequate dosage will be needed to eliminate the infection.

Syphilis

Caused by the corkscrew-shaped (*spirochete*) organism *Treponema pallidum*, syphilis has three phases: primary, secondary, and tertiary.

In the primary phase, there is usually a small, painless sore (*chancre*) on the genitalia which appears ten days to three months after infection. It may, however, be located elsewhere and is sometimes not visible, or even may not appear at all. The only associated symptom may be a mild headache—and this, not always. The chancre will heal on its own in four to six weeks, until which the infected person is highly contagious.

Secondary syphilis appears at or shortly after the time the chancre disappears and is usually manifested by a rash, which sometimes may be fairly widespread, but there is no general feeling of sickness.

The tertiary phase, if syphilis is not treated, occurs years after the primary and secondary phases have gone and can cause brain or heart damage or both, often leading to death.

When should you suspect syphilis? One clue is the appearance of any ulcerlike sore on the genitalia—penis or vulva—particularly if it is painless. And you should be suspicious of any rash or eruption when there are no other symptoms.

A blood test can provide a definitive diagnosis. Treatment is relatively simple: injection of penicillin or use of another antibiotic.

Nonspecific Urethritis

For years, urethritis—inflammation of the urethra, the channel carrying urine from the bladder—has been considered to be synonymous with gonorrhea. This is no longer true. Most clinics in the United States now report that urethritis, in both men and women, results from organisms other than the gonococcus in 40 to 60 percent of cases.

Various organisms can be responsible for what has come to be called nonspecific urethritis. The most common causative agent is *Chlamydia trachomatis*, the same microbe that causes the eye disease trachoma.

In men, symptoms may be mild: pain during urination and a clear, watery mucoid discharge. In women, infection can remain unnoticed in the cervix, producing no apparent symptoms. If untreated, the infection may lead to serious complications. In men, there may be inflammation of the epididymis, which carries sperm from the testis. In women, inflammation may occur in the cervix or fallopian tubes which can become blocked, causing sterility. The infection can be passed on to babies during birth, causing eye infections and pneumonia.

Because a recently developed test for chlamydiae is not yet

widely available, a physician diagnoses nonspecific urethritis by looking for gonococci in a smear or culture of discharge. If none are present, the disease is nonspecific urethritis.

Making the distinction is important, because chlamydiae do not respond to antibiotics such as penicillin, used for gonorrhea. The organisms, however, usually do respond to a tetracycline antibiotic such as Achromycin, Panmycin, or Sumycin. If not, another antibiotic such as erythromycin may be used.

It's essential that a man's sexual partner be examined and, if found to have infection, receive the same treatment. Unless this is done, the disease ping-pongs, recurring among married partners and spreading through the population in other cases.

Genital Herpes

Infection of the genital skin and mucous membranes with a virus, herpesvirus hominis, Type 2 (which belongs to the same family as the virus that causes cold sores), is increasing.

Usually, four to seven days after intercourse, itching and soreness develop before a small, reddened patch appears. A small group of blisterlike lesions develop. The lesions become eroded, producing superficial circular ulcers. The ulcers crust in a few days and usually heal in about ten days with scarring. The ulcers commonly are painful, and there often are enlargement and tenderness of lymph nodes in the groin.

No cure for herpes infection is available. Treatment is symptomatic. The lesions should be kept clean with a salt solution twice a day. Sitz baths may be comforting. A painkiller may be needed.

A relationship exists between herpes infection and cancer of the cervix, but it is not yet completely understood. It could be wise for any woman who has had genital herpes infection to get a Pap smear at regular intervals for life.

There are other venereal diseases—such as lymphogranuloma venereum and granuloma inguinale—but they are rare in the United States.

You are likely to find it difficult to differentiate among the venereal diseases. The safest thing to do is to get a medical examination and appropriate tests if you experience any symptoms affecting areas of sexual contact.

Heterosexual contacts are not the only sources of venereal disease. Most of the diseases can be transmitted through homosexual contacts. Moreover, a recent outbreak of amebic dysentery occurred among homosexual males in California. The disease is caused by an ameba present in the large intestine. It leads to diarrhea, rectal bleeding, and ulceration in the colon. Infection is transmitted by oral and anal contact. Specific antibiotics are available for treatment.

Venous Thrombosis

This condition, which can produce arm or leg swelling and increased warmth of the overlying skin, involves a clot in a vein. You probably have also heard it called *thrombophlebitis, phlebitis, phlebothrombosis,* and *"milk leg."*

Actually, *phlebothrombosis* indicates that little or no inflammation is present with the clot, while *thrombophlebitis* and *phlebitis* indicate definite inflammation of the vein wall. (The ending *-itis* means inflammation; *phleb-* refers to a vein; and *thrombo-* means clot). "Milk leg" is sometimes used to indicate a clot in the iliac or femoral vein with massive leg swelling.

Among the reasons why a clot may form are accidental injury of the lining of a vein and standstill of blood in a vein because of inactivity, prolonged bed rest, or pressure on the back of the leg when sitting in a chair. The clot may grow and, in doing so, may obstruct a vein. The danger of a clot in the leg is that sometimes part or all of it may break loose and be carried in the blood to a lung vessel. If that happens, the clot is called a *pulmonary* (lung) *embolus* (clot that has migrated). On the other hand, the clot may stop enlarging at its original site and become firmly attached there; over a period of some months a new channel for blood flow may form in the vein or new vein branches may develop so blood can detour around the clot.

WHAT TO DO: With venous thrombosis, you should have medical help as soon as possible. Treatment may include elevation of the arm or leg to encourage blood return to the heart, and moist warm packs plus an anticoagulant (anticlotting) drug to prevent further clotting. Elastic stockings are recommended. Usually within five to ten days, tenderness and swelling disappear, and if the leg was affected, you can expect to walk with an elastic support.

Vertigo (See DIZZINESS)

Visceral Larva Migrans (See WORM-INDUCED DISEASES)

Vomiting (See NAUSEA AND VOMITING)

Vomiting Blood (See BLEEDING)

Whipworm (See WORM-INDUCED DISEASES)

Worm-Induced Diseases

Fortunately, many of these diseases have become rare thanks to better control of our water supply and sewage systems. They are not wiped out, however, and some occasionally appear, even sometimes as epidemics, in areas where the water has been contaminated.

Trichinosis

This parasitic disease results from infection with the roundworm *Trichinella spiralis* as a result of eating raw or inadequately cooked or processed pork or pork products.

Many infected people remain free of symptoms. When symptoms occur, they may begin with swelling of the upper eyelids about the eleventh day after infection. This may be followed by bleeding in the eye, eye pain, and sensitivity to light. Diarrhea, nausea, vomiting, and slight fever may precede or accompany the eye symptoms. Muscle soreness and pain, hives, thirst, profuse sweating, chills, weakness, and prostration may follow.

WHAT TO DO: Although there is no specific treatment, trichinosis seldom leads to permanent disability. Muscle pains can be relieved by bed rest and aspirin, or if you consult your physician, he may prescribe codeine. He may also prescribe prednisone or a similar cortisonelike drug for about ten days to relieve other symptoms. The parasites cause no more trouble once they become enclosed in sacs or cysts.

Schistosomiasis

Rare in the United States except among Puerto Ricans, this parasitic disease results from bathing in or other contact with water infested with flukes that penetrate the skin and mature in one to three months into adult worms that invade intestines or bladder.

First symptoms may be fever and hives. Later, dysentery may develop, with markedly fluid stools, cramps, and spasms of involuntary straining to evacuate.

WHAT TO DO: A physician is needed. Among the most effective medications are tartar emetic and stibophen, given by injection, in doses that have to be adjusted carefully; otherwise the drugs may produce upper abdominal pain, dizziness, nausea and vomiting, joint and muscle pain, and heart rate changes.

Visceral Larva Migrans

This is an infection with nematode larvae, which are normal intestinal parasites of pet dogs and cats. Commonly, the infection source is soil or a sandbox contaminated by pet feces containing parasite eggs, which a child may transfer to his mouth while playing. The eggs hatch in the human intestine, and the larvae can penetrate the intestinal wall and get into the circulation, remaining alive for months, producing damage as they move about. They may cause fever, coughing, liver enlargement, lung inflammation.

WHAT TO DO: No specific treatment is available but your physician may prescribe prednisone or a similar cortisonelike drug to help control symptoms. If there is no reinfection, the disease disappears after 6 to 18 months. As a preventive measure against infection or reinfection, infected pets should be dewormed regularly by a veterinarian, and children's sandboxes should be covered when not in use.

Other Intestinal Parasitic Infections

The *giant intestinal roundworm* enters as an egg via contaminated vegetables, producing colicky pains and diarrhea. Diagnosis can be made when immature eggs or worms are found in stools. Among effective medications the physician can prescribe are piperazine, thiabendazole, bephenium hydroxynaphthoate, and hexylresorcinol.

Hookworm may enter via the mouth but more commonly penetrates the skin, usually of the feet. The source of infection is fecal contamination of soil. The worm can cause stools darkened with blood pigments, anemia, retarded growth, heart insufficiency. Mature eggs found in the stool help in diagnosis. The physician can prescribe effective medications, which include tetrachloroethylene, hexylresorcinol, bephenium hydoxynaphthoate, and thiabendazole.

Threadworm, found in the southern United States, enters through the skin, usually of the feet, and the source is fecal contamination of soil. It causes diarrhea and pain in the pit of the stomach which may radiate. Diagnosis is clear when larvae are found in the stool. Effective medication is thiabendazole.

Whipworm, found in the Gulf Coast region, enters as an egg through the mouth. Source is fecal contamination of soil. The infection produces diarrhea, nausea, anemia, retarded growth, and sometimes acute appendicitis in children. Diagnosis is clear when immature eggs are found in the stool. Effective treatment: hexylresorcinol enemas and thiabendazole.

Pinworm enters as an egg through the mouth. Source is a contaminated environment. The infection produces itching around the anal area and often affects an entire family. Diagnosis is clear when eggs are found in anal swabs or adult worms appear. Effective medications the physician can prescribe include piperazine, pyrvinium, pamoate, and thiabendazole.

Dwarf tapeworm, common in children in the southern United States, enters the mouth as an egg from a contaminated environment. Symptoms include diarrhea, abdominal discomfort, dizziness, and inanition (a physical condition like that resulting from starvation). Diagnosis is certain when eggs are found in the stool. Effective medication is quinacrine hydrochloride.

Beef tapeworm enters in larva form from poorly cooked or raw infected beef. It produces abdominal distress and appendicitislike symptoms. Diagnosis can be made when eggs are found in the stool. Effective medication is niclosamide or quinacrine hydrochloride.

Fish tapeworm enters in larva form from infected freshwater fish and may cause pernicious anemia or bowel obstruction. One of the common causes used to be the preparation of gefilte fish by Jewish women at home; they would taste the raw fish patties before cooking. Diagnosis of fish tapeworm can be made when immature eggs are found in the stool. Effective medication is niclosamide.

Amebic dysentery is caused by *Entamoeba histolytica,* a protozoan, which enters via the mouth from feces-contaminated water, food, and the environment. It causes attacks of diarrhea over a prolonged period and may produce complications such as liver and lung abscesses. Diagnosis can be made when the organism is found in the stool. Effective medication includes emetine hydrochloride, tetracycline, metronidazole, and chloroquine phosphate.

Giardia is a parasitic protozoan that enters as a cyst through the mouth. Source is contaminated human feces. The infection produces mucous diarrhea, abdominal pain, and weight loss. Diagnosis is certain when the organism is found in the stool. Effective medication includes quinacrine hydrochloride and metronidazole.

Wounds, Puncture

A puncture wound may be caused by a nail, tack, pin, or other sharp object.

WHAT TO DO: Because puncture wounds often do not bleed freely and contamination may be sealed in, gently press around the wound (do not squeeze) to encourage bleeding. If the wound should bleed spontaneously, let it bleed enough to wash out any contamination, unless gushing blood indicates injury to an artery; in that case, apply pressure.

After washing your hands thoroughly, check to make certain that no foreign object is left in the wound (a broken-off part of a needle, for example). If there is a foreign body, remove if possible. If you cannot, a physician must see the wound.

Clean around the wound with soap and warm water. If hydrogen peroxide is available, it can also be used for cleansing.

Cover the wound with sterile dressing.

Thereafter, warm-water soaks can be used several times a day for several days to keep the puncture open so any microorganisms and debris can drain.

Even if the wound is minor, check with your physician by phone about whether an antibiotic may be needed or a tetanus shot.

Tetanus always has to be considered. Protection against it in the form of injection may or may not be needed, depending upon the nature and extent of the wound and your immunization status or lack of it. Let your physician decide.

If bacterial infection develops, the indications will not come for about 24 hours and then will consist of pus, fever, or severe swelling and redness. The physician should then see the wound.

It's advisable to see a physician when there is a puncture wound of the chest, abdomen, or head—unless it is clearly a minor wound—because of the possibility of internal injury.

If blood gushes from the wound (indicating injury to an artery) or if numbness or tingling is experienced (indicating injury to a nerve), a physician should be seen.

Any deep puncture wound of the hand may lead to infection which, once it takes hold, may be difficult to combat. For this reason, a physician should be called about the advisability of preventive antibiotic treatment.

Part Three

A Guide to Acute Emergency Reactions from Drugs

Almost anything taken into the human body can, in some people, produce an undesirable reaction.

That, of course, is true even of foods, some of which, although enjoyed without penalty by most people, can produce for a small minority reactions that may range from outbreaks of hives or skin wheals to gastrointestinal distress.

It is no less true of drugs, including the most valued of prescription drugs.

To follow is a listing of symptoms that sometimes can occur as reactions to prescription medications.

A second listing presents the drugs in alphabetical order according to trade name and also shows the generic name of each and its major uses.

If there is any possibility that some medication recently prescribed for you may be causing trouble, call your physician and discuss it with him. Not infrequently, undesirable side reactions develop early in the course of taking a medication and then disappear with continued use. In other cases, the reactions will continue unless measures are taken to counter them. The measures can include a change of dosage or a switch to another medication, equally useful, which may not produce an undesirable reaction for you. If a drug is vital and there is no substitute for it, it is often possible to neutralize an undesirable effect with additional medication.

Acute Reactions and the Drugs That May Produce Them

Abdominal disturbances. Aldactazide, Aldactone, Aldoril, Ambenyl Expectorant, Aristocort, Atromid-S, Azo Gantrisin, Benadryl, Butazolidin, Butazolidin Alka, Cleocin, Coumadin, Cyclospasmol, Darvon, Decadron, Demulen, Dimetapp, Diuril, Drixoral, E-Mycin, Erythrocin, Erythromycin, Esidrix, Gantanol, Gantrisin, Hydrodiuril, Hygroton, Inderal, Indocin, Kaon, Keflex, Lomotil, Macrodantin, Medrol, Norlestrin preparations, Oracon preparations, Ornade,

Ortho-Novum preparations, Ovral, Ovulen 21, Pavabid, Pediamycin, penicillin G potassium, Penicillin VK, Pentids, Pen-Vee K, Periactin, Premarin, Rauzide, Ritalin, Salutensin, Sterazolidin, Sumycin, Talwin, Tandearil, Tenuate, Terramycin, tetracycline, Tetrex, Tofranil, Tuss-Ornade, V-Cillin K, Zyloprim.

Agitation. Butazolidin, Butazolidin Alka, Compazine, Demerol, Mellaril, Stelazine, Sterazolidin, Tandearil, Tofranil, Triavil.

Allergic reactions. Combid, Nembutal, Neosporin, phenobarbital, Seconal.

Anaphylaxis. Amcill, ampicillin, Declomycin, Dimetane, Diupres, Dyazide, E-Mycin, Equanil, Erythrocin, Erythromycin, Etrafon, Macrodantin, Mellaril, Minocin, Omnipen, Parafon Forte, Pediamycin, Penbritin, penicillin G potassium, Penicillin VK, Pentids, Pen-Vee K, Periactin, Polycillin, Principen, Stelazine, Sumycin, Terramycin, tetracycline, Tetrex, V-Cillin K, Vibramycin.

Angioneurotic edema (giant hives). Declomycin, Equanil, Etrafon, Lomotil, Macrodantin, Mellaril, Minocin, Mysteclin-F, Parafon Forte, Sumycin, Terramycin, tetracycline, Tetrex, Tuinal, Vibramycin.

Anogenital itching/irritation. Minocin, Sumycin, Terramycin, tetracycline, Tetrex, Valium, Vibramycin.

Backache. Norlestrin preparations, Oracon preparations, Ortho-Novum preparations, Ovral, Ovulen 21.

Bleeding, gastrointestinal. Butazolidin, Butazolidin Alka, Indocin, Parafon Forte, Sterazolidin, Tandearil.

Breathing difficulty. Aldoril, Apresoline, Diupres, Hydrodiuril, Hydropres, Inderal, Indocin, Macrodantin, quinidine sulfate, Rauzide, reserpine, Salutensin, Ser-Ap-Es.

Bruising. Aldactazide, Aldoril, Hydrodiuril, Medrol.

Chest pain. Apresoline, Dalmane, Diupres, Drixoral, Hydropres, Macrodantin, Marex, Ornade, Proloid, Rauzide, Regroton, reserpine, Ritalin, Salutensin, Ser-Ap-Es, Tenuate, thyroid, Tuss-Ornade.

Chest tightness. Ambenyl Expectorant, Benadryl, Dimetane, Dimetapp, Ornade, Periactin, Tuss-Ornade.

Chills. Apresoline, Azo Gantrisin, Equanil, Gantanol, Gantrisin, Macrodantin, meprobamate, penicillin G potassium, Penicillin VK, Pentids, Pen-Vee K, Sinequan, Talwin, V-Cillin K.

Confusion. Aldactazide, Aldactone, Ambenyl Expectorant, Benadryl, Butazolidin, Butazolidin Alka, Dalmane, Dilantin, Dimetane, Drixoral, Elavil, Etrafon, Indocin, Kaon, Librax, Librium, Mellaril, Norgesic, Periactin, quinidine sulfate, Sinequan, Sterazolidin, Tandearil, Tofranil, Tranxene, Triavil, Valium.

Constipation. Aldomet, Aldoril, Ambenyl Expectorant, Apresoline, Artane, Benadryl, Bendectin, Bentyl, Bentyl/phenobarbital, Combid, Dalmane, Darvon preparations, Demerol, Dilantin, Dimetane, Dimetapp, Diupres, Diuril, Dyazide, Elavil, Esidrix, Etrafon, Feosol, Fiorinal, Fiorinal/codeine, Hydrodiuril, Hygroton, Inderal, Ionamin, Librax, Librium, Mellaril, Norgesic, Ornade, Pavabid, Percodan, Phenaphen/codeine, Pro-Banthine, Rauzide, Regroton, Salutensin, Ser-Ap-Es, Sinequan, Stelazine, Talwin, Tenuate, Thorazine, Tofranil, Triavil, Valium.

Convulsions. Aristocort, Atarax, Azo Gantrisin, Combid, Decadron, Gantanol, Gantrisin, Garamycin, Medrol, Ornade, prednisone, Sterazolidin, Tandearil, Thorazine, Tigan, Tuss-Ornade, Vistaril.

Depression. Aldomet, Aldoril, Apresoline, Azo Gantrisin, Demulen, Diupres, Gantanol, Gantrisin, Hydropres, Inderal, Indocin, Lomotil, Norlestrin preparations, Oracon preparations, Ortho-Novum preparations, Ovral, Ovulen 21, Rauzide, Regroton, reserpine, Ser-Ap-Es, Tenuate, Valium.

Diarrhea. Aldactazide, Aldactone, Aldomet, Aldoril, Ambenyl Expectorant, Amcill, ampicillin, Apresoline, Atromid-S, Azo Gantrisin, Benadryl, Bendectin, Butazolidin, Butazolidin Alka, Cleocin, Coumadin, Dalmane, Declomycin, Diabinese, Dimetane, Dimetapp, Diupres, Diuril, Dyazide, Elavil, E-Mycin, Equanil, Erythrocin, Erythromycin, Esidrix, Feosol, Gantanol, Gantrisin, Hydrodiuril, Hydropres, Hygroton, Inderal, Indocin, Ionamin, Kaon, Keflex, Lanoxin, Lasix, Macrodantin, Mellaril, meprobamate, Minocin, Mycostatin, Mysteclin-F, Noludar, Omnipen, Ornade, Pavabid, Pediamycin, Penbritin, penicillin

G potasium, Penicillin VK, Pentids, Pen-Vee K, Polycillin, Principen, Rauzide, Regroton, reserpine, Salutensin, Ser-Ap-Es, Sinequan, Sterazolidin, Talwin, Tandearil, Terramycin, tetracycline, Tetrex, Tigan, Tofranil, Triavil, Tuss-Ornade, Vibramycin, V-Cillin K, Zyloprim.

Dizziness/vertigo. Aldactazide, Aldomet, Aldoril, Ambenyl Expectorant, Apresoline, Aristocort, Artane, Atromid-S, Azo Gantrisin, Benadryl, Bendectin, Bentyl, Bentyl/phenobarbital, Butazolidin, Butazolidin Alka, Chlor-Trimeton, Combid, Compazine, Dalmane, Darvon preparations, Decadron, Demerol, Dilantin, Dimetane, Dimetapp, Diupres, Diuril, Drixoral, Dyazide, Elavil, Equanil, Esidrix, Etrafon, Fiorinal, Fiorinal/codeine, Gantanol, Gantrisin, Garamycin, Hydropres, Hygroton, Indocin, Ionamin, Isordil, Keflex, Lasix, Lomotil, Macrodantin, Marex, Medrol, meprobamate, nitroglycerin, Noludar, Norgesic, Norlestrin preparations, Oracon preparations, Ornade, Ortho-Novum preparations, Ovral, Ovulen 21, Parafon Forte, Pavabid, Percodan, Periactin, Peritrate, Phenergan preparations, Placidyl, Polaramine, prednisone, Pro-Banthine, quinidine sulfate, Rauzide, Regroton, reserpine, Ritalin, Salutensin, Ser-Ap-Es, Serax, Sinequan, Stelazine, Sterazolidin, Sumycin, Talwin, Teldrin, Tenuate, Terramycin, tetracycline, Tetrex, Thorazine, Tofranil, Tolinase, Tranxene, Triaminic, Triavil, Tuss-Ornade, Valium, Vasodilan.

Dyspepsia. Atromid-S, Butazolidin, Butazolidin Alka, Keflex, Sinequan, Sterazolidin, Tandearil.

Ear ringing. Azo Gantrisin, Dimetane, Dimetapp, Elavil, Gantanol, Gantrisin, Garamycin, Lasix, Periactin, Sinequan, Talwin, Triavil.

Edema (fluid accumulation). Aldomet, Aldoril, Apresoline, Aristocort, Butazolidin, Butazolidin Alka, Combid, Decadron, Demulen, Diabinese, Diupres, Etrafon, Librax, Librium, Medrol, Norlestrin preparations, Oracon preparations, Ortho-Novum preparations, Ovral, Ovulen 21, penicillin G potassium, Penicillin VK, Pentids, Pen-Vee K, prednisone, Premarin, quinidine sulfate, Salutensin, Serax, Sinequan, Stelazine, Sterazolidin, Tandearil, Tofranil, Triavil, V-Cillin K.

Eye disturbances. Apresoline, Azo Gantrisin, Dalmane, Gantanol, Gantrisin, Indocin, Norlestrin preparations, Oracon preparations, Ortho-Novum preparations, Ovral, Ovulen 21, Thorazine.

Faintness. Dalmane, Demerol, Dimetapp, Diupres, Equanil, Hydropres, Indocin, Librax, Librium, meprobamate, nitroglycerin, Periactin, Salutensin, Ser-Ap-Es, Serax, Talwin, Thorazine.

Fever. Aldactazide, Aldactone, Aldoril, Apresoline, Azo Gantrisin, Butazolidin, Butazolidin Alka, Combid, Coumadin, Diabinese, Diuril, Equanil, Gantanol, Gantrisin, Garamycin, Hydrodiuril, Inderal, Macrodantin, Mellaril, meprobamate, Mysteclin-F, penicillin G potassium, Penicillin VK, Pentids, Pen-Vee K, quinidine sulfate, Ritalin, Serax, Stelazine, Sterazolidin, Sumycin, Tandearil, Terramycin, tetracycline, Tetrex, Thorazine, thyroid, Tofranil, V-Cillin K, Zyloprim.

Flatulence (gas). Aldomet, Aldoril, Atromid-S.

Gastrointestinal upset. Mycostatin, nicotinic acid, Pyridium, Parafon Forte, quinidine sulfate, Tranxene, Triaminic.

Hallucinations. Azo Gantrisin, Dalmane, Demerol, Elavil, Gantanol, Gantrisin, Inderal, Periactin, Serax, Sinequan, Talwin, Triavil.

Headache. Afrin, Aldactazide, Aldomet, Aldoril, Ambenyl Expectorant, Apresoline, Aristocort, Artane, Atromid-S, Azo Gantrisin, Benadryl, Bendectin, Bentyl, Bentyl/phenobarbital, Butazolidin, Butazolidin Alka, Butisol Sodium, Chlor-Trimeton, Combid, Cyclospasmol, Dalmane, Darvon preparations, Decadron, Demerol, Demulen, Dilantin, Dimetane, Dimetapp, Diupres, Diuril, Drixoral, Dyazide, Equanil, Esidrix, Etrafon, Gantanol, Gantrisin, Garamycin, Hydrodiuril, Hydropres, Hygroton, Indocin, Ionamin, Isordil, Keflex, Lanoxin, Lasix, Lomotil, Macrodantin, Marax, Medrol, Mellaril, meprobamate, nicotinic acid, nitroglycerin, Noludar, Norgesic, Orinase, Ornade, Pavabid, Periactin, Polaramine, prednisone, Premarin, Pro-Banthine, quinidine sulfate, Rauzide, Regroton, reserpine, Ritalin, Salutensin, Ser-Ap-Es, Serax, Stelazine, Sterazolidin, Sumycin, Talwin, Tandearil, Tenuate, Terramycin, tetracycline, Tetrex, thyroid, Tofranil, Tolinase, Tranxene, Tuss-Ornade, Valium.

Hearing impairment. Aristocort, Butazolidin, Butazolidin Alka, Decadron, Diupres, Hydropres, Indocin, Lasix, quinidine sulfate, Regroton, reserpine, Salutensin, Ser-Ap-Es, Sterazolidin, Tandearil.

Heartbeat, fast. Apresoline, Bentyl, Bentyl/phenobarbital, Cyclospasmol, Demerol, Dimetane, Teldrin, Tenuate, Thorazine, thyroid, Tofranil.

Heartbeat, slow. Aldomet, Aldoril, Demerol.

Heartburn. Chlor-Trimeton, Cyclospasmol, Dalmane, Etrafon, Orinase, Polaramine.

Heart rhythm disturbances. Elavil, Hydropres, Kaon, Lanoxin, Marax, Proloid, Rauzide, reserpine, Ritalin, Ser-Ap-Es, Tenuate, Tofranil, Triavil.

Hives. Achromycin V, Aldactazide, Aldactone, Aldoril, Ambenyl Expectorant, Amcill, ampicillin, Apresoline, Atromid-S, Azo Gantrisin, Benadryl, Bentyl, Bentyl/phenobarbital, Butazolidin, Butazolidin Alka, Cleocin, Coumadin, Declomycin, Demerol, Dimetane, Dimetapp, Diuril, Dyazide, Elavil, E-Mycin, Erythrocin, Erythromycin, Esidrix, Etrafon, Gantanol, Gantrisin, Garamycin, Hydrodiuril, Hygroton, Indocin, Ionamin, Keflex, Lasix, Lomotil, Macrodantin, Minocin, Mysteclin-F, Norgesic, Omnipen, Omnipres, Orinase, Pediamycin, Penbritin, penicillin G potassium, Penicillin VK, Pentids, Pen-Vee K, Periactin, Placidyl, Polycillin, Principen, Rauzide, Regroton, Ritalin, Salutensin, Ser-Ap-Es, Stelazine, Sterazolidin, Sumycin, Talwin, Tandearil, Terramycin, tetracycline, Tetrex, Thorazine, Tofranil, Tolinase, Triavil, Tuinal, Vibramycin, Zyloprim.

Hoarseness. Sumycin, Terramycin, tetracycline, Tetrex.

Insomnia. Afrin, Ambenyl Expectorant, Azo Gantrisin, Benadryl, Bentyl, Bentyl/phenobarbital, Butazolidin, Butazolidin Alka, Compazine, Dilantin, Dimetane, Drixoral, Elavil, Etrafon, Gantanol, Gantrisin, Ionamin, Marax, Ornade, Periactin, Pro-Banthine, Ritalin, Stelazine, Talwin, Tedral, Tenuate, thyroid, Tofranil, Tranxene, Triavil, Tuss-Ornade, Valium.

Irritability. Benedectin, Dalmane, Ornade, Tranxene, Tuss-Ornade.

Itching. Aldactazide, Apresoline, Atromid-S, Azo Gantrisin, Combid, Cordran, Dalmane, Demerol, Diupres, Etrafon, Gantanol, Gantrisin, Garamycin, Indocin, Keflex, Kenalog, Lomotil, Lasix, Macrodantin, Mycolog, Mysteclin-F, nicotinic acid, Norlestrin preparations, Oracon preparations, Orinase, Ortho-Nóvum preparations, Ovral, Ovulen 21, Percodan, Regroton, reserpine, Salutensin, Ser-Ap-Es, Sinequan, Stelazine, Synalar, Valisone, Vioform-Hydrocortisone, Zyloprim.

Jaundice. Aldactazide, Aldoril, Cleocin, Combid, Compazine, Demulen, Diabinese, Diupres, Diuril, Elavil, Esidrix, Etrafon, Hydrodiuril, Hygroton, Indocin, Lasix, Macrodantin, Mellaril, nicotinic acid, Norlestrin preparations, Oracon preparations, Orinase, Ortho-Novum preparations, Ovral, Ovulen 21, Parafon Forte, Placidyl, Rauzide, Regroton, Salutensin, Ser-Ap-Es, Serax, Sinequan, Stelazine, Thorazine, Tigan, Tofranil, Tolinase, Triavil, Valium.

Joint pain. Aldomet, Aldoril, Apresoline, Atromid-S, Azo Gantrisin, Butazolidin, Butazolidin Alka, Dalmane, Gantanol, Gantrisin, Macrodantin, Mysteclin-F, penicillin G potassium, Penicillin VK, Pentids, Pen-Vee K, Ritalin, Ser-Ap-Es, Sterazolidin, Sumycin, Tandearil, Terramycin, Tetracycline, Tetrex, Valium, V-Cillin K, Zyloprim.

Light-headedness. Afrin, Aldomet, Aldoril, Dalmane, Darvon preparations, Demerol, Indocin, Lasix, Parafon Forte, Percodan, Talwin.

Malaise. Lomotil, Macrodantin, Pavabid, Percodan, Tenuate, Tolinase.

Menstrual irregularities. Aldactazide, Aldactone, Aristocort, Combid, Decadron, Demulen, Etrafon, Librax, Librium, Medrol, Mellaril, prednisone, Proloid (overdose), Serax, Stelazine, Sterazolidin, Tenuate.

Migraine. Norlestrin preparations, Oracon preparations, Ortho-Novum preparations, Ovral, Ovulen 21, Premarin.

Miliaria (prickly heat). Cordran, Kenalog, Mycolog, Synalar, Valisone.

Mouth dryness. Aldomet, Aldoril, Ambenyl Expectorant,

Antivert, Artane, Atarax, Bellergal, Benadryl, Bendectin, Bentyl, Bentyl/phenobarbital, Chlor-Trimeton, Combid, Dalmane, Demerol, Dimetane, Donnagel-PG, Donnatal, Diupres, Dyazide, Etrafon, Hydropres, Ionamin, Librax, Librium, Mellaril, Norgesic, Ornade, Phenergan preparations, Pro-Banthine, Polaramine, Rauzide, Regroton, reserpine, Salutensin, Ser-Ap-Es, Sinequan, Stelazine, Teldrin, Tenuate, Thorazine, Tofranil, Tranxene, Tuss-Ornade, Vistaril.

Mouth inflammation. Amcill, ampicillin, Azo Gantrisin, Indocin, Mysteclin-F, Omnipen, Penbritin, Polycillin, Principen, Sumycin, Terramycin, tetracycline, Tetrex, Tofranil, Vibramycin.

Muscle ache. Atromid-S, Diupres, Hydropres, Rauzide, Regroton, reserpine, Salutensin, Ser-Ap-Es.

Muscle cramps. Apresoline, Atromid-S, Dyazide, Lasix, Regroton, Ser-Ap-Es, Tigan.

Muscle pain. Aldomet, Aldoril, phenobarbital, Tenuate.

Muscle spasm. Aldoril, Compazine, Diupres, Diuril, Esidrix, Hydrodiuril, Hygroton, Rauzide, Salutensin, Stelazine, Triavil.

Muscle weakness. Aristocort, Atromid-S, Decadron, Marax, Medrol, prednisone, Stelazine, Sterazolidin.

Nasal congestion. Afrin, Apresoline, Combid, Diupres, Etrafon, Hydropres, Regroton, reserpine, Ser-Ap-Es, Salutensin, Stelazine, Thorazine.

Nasal dryness. Afrin, Ambenyl Expectorant, Benadryl, Dimetane, Marax, Ornade, Tuss-Ornade.

Nasal stuffiness. Aldomet, Aldoril, Ambenyl Expectorant, Benadryl, Dimetane, Mellaril.

Nausea/vomiting. Achromycin V, Aldactazide, Aldomet, Aldoril, Ambenyl Expectorant, Amcill, ampicillin, Apresoline, Artane, Atromid-S, Azo Gantrisin, Benadryl, Bendectin, Bentyl, Bentyl/phenobarbital, Butisol Sodium, Butazolidin, Butazolidin Alka, Cleocin, Coumadin, Dalmane, Darvon preparations, Declomycin, Demerol, Demulen, Dilantin, Dimetapp, Diabinese, Diupres, Diuril, Doriden, Drixoral, Dyazide, Elavil, E-Mycin, Equanil, Erythrocin, Erythromycin, Esidrix, Etrafon, Feosol, Fiorinal, Fiorinal/codeine, Gantanol, Gantrisin, Garamycin, Hydergine, Hydrodiuril,

Hydropres, Hygroton, Inderal, Indocin, Isordil, Kaon, Keflex, Lanoxin, Lasix, Librax, Librium, Lomotil, Macrodantin, Marax, meprobamate, Mellaril, Minocin, Mycostatin, Mysteclin-F, Nembutal, Noludar, Norgesic, Norlestrin preparations, Omnipen, Oracon preparations, Orinase, Ornade, Ortho-Novum preparations, Ovral, Ovulen 21, Pavabid, Pediamycin, Penbritin, penicillin G potassium, Penicillin VK, Pentids, Pen-Vee K, Percodan, Periactin, Peritrate, Phenergan/codeine, Placidyl, Polaramine, Polycillin, Premarin, Pro-Banthine, quinidine sulfate, Rauzide, Regroton, Salutensin, Ser-Ap-Es, Serax, Sinequan, Stelazine, Sterazolidin, Sumycin, Talwin, Tandearil, Tenuate, Terramycin, tetracycline, Tetrex, thyroid, Tofranil, Tolinase, Triavil, Tuss-Ornade, Valium, V-Cillin K, Vibramycin, Zyloprim.

Nervousness. Ambenyl Expectorant, Artane, Bentyl, Bentyl/phenobarbital, Dalmane, Dilantin, Dimetane, Diupres, Hydropres, Marax, Norlestrin preparations, Oracon preparations, Ornade, Ortho-Novum preparations, Ovral, Ovulen 21, Periactin, Polaramine, Pro-Banthine, Proloid (overdose), Rauzide, Ritalin, Salutensin, Ser-Ap-Es, Tenuate, thyroid (overdose), Tranxene, Triaminic, Tuss-Ornade.

Nightmares. Aldomet, Aldoril, Diupres, Elavil, Hydropres, Regroton, reserpine, Salutensin, Ser-Ap-Es, Tofranil, Triavil.

Nosebleed. Indocin, Salutensin, Ser-Ap-Es.

Numbness. Apresoline, Elavil, Etrafon, Garamycin, Lomotil, Ser-Ap-Es, Talwin, Tofranil, Triavil.

Palpitation. Afrin, Ambenyl Expectorant, Apresoline, Benadryl, Bendectin, Bentyl, Bentyl/phenobarbital, Dalmane, Demerol, Dimetane, Dimetapp, Drixoral, Elavil, Equanil, Etrafon, Ionamin, Marax, meprobamate, nitroglycerin, Norgesic, Ornade, Periactin, Ritalin, Ser-Ap-Es, Tedral, Tenuate, Tofranil, Triaminic, Triavil, Tuss-Ornade, Vasodilan.

Pulse, fast. Elavil, Equanil, Ionamin, meprobamate, nitroglycerin, Norgesic, Triavil.

Restlessness. Aldactazide, Aldoril, Ambenyl Expectorant, Benadryl, Chlor-Trimeton, Dalmane, Darvon preparations, Demerol, Dimetane, Diupres, Diuril, Drixoral, Elavil, Esidrix, Hydrodiuril, Hygroton, Ionamin, Isordil, Lomotil, Mellaril, Percodan, Periactin, Peritrate, Polaramine, Regroton, Salutensin, Ser-Ap-Es, Tenuate, Tofranil, Triavil.

Seizures (see also Convulsions). Elavil, Etrafon, Tofranil, Triavil.

Skin rash or eruption. Achromycin V, Aldactazide, Aldactone, Aldomet, Aldoril, Ambenyl Expectorant, Amcill, ampicillin, Apresoline, Atromid-S, Azo Gantrisin, Benadryl, Bendectin, Butazolidin, Butazolidin Alka, Butisol Sodium, Cleocin, Coumadin, Dalmane, Darvon preparations, Declomycin, Demerol, Demulen, Dilantin, Dimetane, Dimetapp, Diupres, Diuril, Doriden, Drixoral, Dyazide, Elavil, E-Mycin, Equanil, Erythrocin, Erythromycin, Esidrix, Etrafon, Fiorinal, Fiorinal/codeine, Gantrisin, Garamycin, Hydrodiuril, Hygroton, Inderal, Indocin, Isordil, Keflex, Kenalog, Lasix, Librax, Librium, Macrodantin, Mellaril, meprobamate, Minocin, Mycolog, Mysteclin-F, Nembutal, Norgesic, Norlestrin preparations, Omnipen, Oracon preparations, Orinase, Ornade, Ortho-Novum preparations, Ovral, Ovulen 21, Parafon Forte, Pavabid, Pediamycin, Penbritin, penicillin G potassium, Penicillin VK, Pentids, Pen-Vee K, Periactin, Peritrate, phenobarbital, Polaramine, Polycillin, Premarin, Principen, Pro-Banthine, quinidine sulfate, Rauzide, Regroton, reserpine, Ritalin, Salutensin, Ser-Ap-Es, Serax, Sinequan, Stelazine, Sterazolidin, Sumycin, Synalar, Talwin, Tandearil, Tenuate, Terramycin, tetracycline, Tetrex, Thorazine, Tigan, Tofranil, Tolinase, Tranxene, Triavil, Tuss-Ornade, Valisone, Valium, Vasodilan, V-Cillin K, Vibramycin, Vioform-Hydrocortisone, Zyloprim.

Swallowing difficulty. Combid, Compazine, Declomycin, Minocin, Mysteclin-F, Stelazine, Sumycin, Terramycin, tetracycline, Tetrex, Triavil, Vibramycin.

Sweating. Aristocort, Dalmane, Decadron, Demerol, Drixoral, Isordil, Lasix, Marax, Medrol, Pavabid, Peritrate, Polaramine, prednisone, Sterazolidin, Talwin, thyroid, Tofranil.

Throat, sore. Inderal, Mysteclin-F, Tofranil.

Tingling. Aldactazide, Aldomet, Aldoril, Ambenyl Expectorant, Apresoline, Elavil, Equanil, Esidrix, Etrafon, Garamycin, Hydrodiuril, Hygroton, Inderal, Kaon, Lasix, meprobamate, Ser-Ap-Es, Sinequan, Talwin, Tofranil, Triavil.

Tongue, black/hairy. Amcill, ampicillin, Elavil, Mysteclin-F, Omnipen, Penbritin, penicillin G potassium, Penicillin VK, Pentids, Pen Vee K, Polycillin, Principen, Sumycin, Terramycin, tetracycline, Tetrex, Tofranil, Triavil, V-Cillin K.

Tongue inflammation. Amcill, ampicillin, Declomycin, Mysteclin-F, Minocin, Omnipen, Penbritin, Polycillin, Principen.

Tongue, sore. Aldomet, Aldoril, Amcill, ampicillin, Omnipen, Polycillin.

Ulcer, gastrointestinal (esophagus, stomach, or duodenum). Aristocort, Butazolidin, Butazolidin Alka, Decadron, Indocin, Medrol, nicotinic acid, prednisone, Sterazolidin, Tandearil.

Urinary hesitancy. Bentyl, Bentyl/phenobarbital, Combid, Librax, Librium, Marax, Norgesic.

Urinary incontinence. Etrafon, Mellaril, Valium.

Urination, difficult. Apresoline, Benadryl, Dimetane, Donnagel-PG, Donnatal, Ornade, Periactin, Ser-Ap-Es, Tedral, Tuss-Ornade.

Urination, diminished. Azo Gantrisin, Equanil, Gantanol, Gantrisin, Garamycin, meprobamate.

Urination, excessive. Chlor-Trimeton, Polaramine, Tenuate.

Urination, frequent. Dimetane, Dimetapp, Elavil, Etrafon, Periactin, Triavil.

Urination, painful. Bendectin, Chlor-Trimeton, Dimetapp, Drixoral, Ornade, Polaramine, Rauzide, Regroton, Salutensin, Ser-Ap-Es, Tenuate, Tuss-Ornade.

Urine retention. Bentyl, Bentyl/phenobarbital, Combid, Demerol, Dimetane, Elavil, Etrafon, Marax, Mellaril, Norgesic, Periactin, Sinequan, Talwin, Thorazine, Tofranil, Triavil, Valium.

Vaginal bleeding. Indocin.

Vaginal discharge. Keflex.

Vision blurring. Aldoril, Ambenyl Expectorant, Antivert, Artane, Bellergal, Benadryl, Bendectin, Bentyl, Bentyl/phenobarbital, Butazolidin, Butazolidin Alka, Combid,

Compazine, Dalmane, Dimetane, Donnagel-PG, Donnatal, Diupres, Diuril, Doriden, Elavil, Etrafon, Hydrodiuril, Indocin, Lanoxin, Lasix, Librax, Librium, Mellaril, Norgesic, Periactin, Phenergan preparations, Placidyl, Pro-Banthine, Regroton, reserpine, Salutensin, Serax, Sinequan, Stelazine, Sterazolidin, Talwin, Tandearil, Tigan, Tofranil, Tranxene, Triaminic, Triavil.

Vision, double. Ambenyl Expectorant, Benadryl, Dimetane, Periactin, Polaramine, Serax.

Vomiting blood. Butazolidin, Butazolidin Alka, Sterazolidin, Tandearil.

Wheezing. Ambenyl Expectorant, Dimetane, Periactin.

Drugs That May Produce Acute Reactions
Trade name (generic name) and uses

Achromycin V (tetracycline). For infection.

Afrin (oxymetazoline). For nasal congestion.

Aldactazide (spironolactone and hydrochlorothiazide). For edema, high blood pressure.

Aldactone (spironolactone). For edema, high blood pressure.

Aldomet (methyldopa). For high blood pressure.

Aldoril (methyldopa and hydrochlorothiazide). For high blood pressure.

Ambenyl Expectorant (codeine, bromodiphenhydramine, diphenhydramine, ammonium chloride, potassium guaiacolsulfonate, menthol). For cough.

Amcill (ampicillin). Semisynthetic penicillin for infection.

Ampicillin. Semisynthetic penicillin for infection.

Antivert (meclizine). For motion sickness, vertigo from ear disturbances.

Apresoline (hydralazine). For high blood pressure.

Aristocort (triamicinolone). For allergies, arthritic conditions, some skin disorders.

Artane (trihexyphenidyl). For Parkinson's disease and control of some nervous system side effects of tranquilizers.

Atarax (hydroxyzine). For anxiety, tension.

Atromid-S (clofibrate). For reducing elevated blood-fat levels.

Azo Gantrisin (sulfamethoxazole and phenazopyridine). For painful urinary infections.

Bellergal (phenobarbital, belladonna, ergotamine tartrate). For menopausal symptoms, premenstrual tension, recurrent throbbing headache, nervous stomach, uterine cramps, some heart conditions.

Benadryl (diphenhydramine). For allergy, motion sickness, insomnia.

Bendectin (dicyclomine, doxylamine, pyridoxine). For nausea and vomiting of pregnancy.

Bentyl (dicyclomine). For irritable bowel, intestinal inflammation.

Bentyl/phenobarbital (dicyclomine, phenobarbital). For irritable bowel, intestinal inflammation.

Butazolidin and Butazolidin Alka (phenylbutazone). For arthritic conditions, gout, painful shoulder.

Butisol Sodium (butabarbital). For sedation, sleep.

Chlor-Trimeton (chlorpheniramine maleate). For allergy.

Cleocin (clindamycin). For infection.

Combid (prochlorperazine, isopropamide). For peptic ulcer, irritable bowel, diarrhea.

Compazine (prochlorperazine). For severe nausea, excessive anxiety, tension, agitation.

Cordran (flurandrenolide). For inflammatory skin conditions.

Coumadin (warfarin). For venous thrombosis, pulmonary embolism, heartbeat irregularity (atrial fibrillation), coronary occlusion.

Cyclospasmol (cyclandelate). For intermittent claudication, thrombophlebitis, Raynaud's disease, nocturnal leg cramps, and some other blood vessel disorders.

Dalmane (flurazepam). For insomnia.

Darvon (propoxyphene); Darvon Compound 65 (with aspirin, phenacetin, caffeine); Darvon N/ASA (with aspirin); Darvocet-N (with acetaminophen). For mild to moderate pain.

Decadron (dexamethasone). For endocrine disorders, arthritis, bursitis, some severe allergic, skin, eye, intestinal, respiratory, blood, and malignant diseases.

Declomycin (demeclocycline).   For infection.
Demerol (meperidine).   Narcotic analgesic for pain.
Demulen (ethynodiol, ethinyl).   Oral contraceptive.
Diabinese (chlorpropamide).   For diabetes.
Dilantin (phenytoin).   For epilepsy.
Dimetane (brompheniramine).   For allergy.
Dimetapp (brompheniramine, phenylephrine, phenylpropa-
nolamine).   Decongestant for allergy.
Diupres (chlorothiazide, reserpine).   For high blood pres-
sure.
Diuril (chlorothiazide).   For edema, high blood pressure, tox-
emia of pregnancy.
Donnagel-PG (kaolin, pectin, hyoscyamine, atropine, hyo-
scine).   For diarrhea.
Donnatal   (hyoscyamine,   atropine,   hyoscine,   pheno-
barbital).   For digestive disorders, gallbladder inflam-
mation, urinary frequency, painful menstruation, premen-
strual tension, motion sickness.
Doriden (glutethimide).   Nonbarbiturate sleeping medica-
tion.
Drixoral (dexbrompheniramine, *d*-isoephedrine).   For nasal
congestion.
Dyazide (triamterene, hydrochlorothiazide).   For edema,
high blood pressure.
Elavil (amitriptyline).   For mental depression.
E-Mycin (erythromycin).   For infection.
Equanil (meprobamate).   For anxiety, tension.
Erythrocin (erythromycin).   For infection.
Erythromycin.   For infection.
Esidrix (hydroclorothiazide).   For high blood pressure,
edema, toxemia of pregnancy.
Etrafon (perphenazine, amitriptyline).   For anxiety, agita-
tion, mental depression.
Feosol (ferrous sulfate).   For iron deficiency and iron-defi-
ciency anemia.
Fiorinal (butalbitol, caffeine, aspirin, phenacetin).   For head-
ache, other pain.
Fiorinal/codeine (Fiorinal plus codeine).   For pain, cough.
Gantanol (sulfamethoxazole).   For urinary and other infec-
tion.

Gantrisin (sulfisoxazole). For urinary and other infection.

Garamycin (gentamicin). For infection.

Hydergine (dihydroergocornine, dihydroergocristine, dihydroergocryptine). For mood depression, confusion, unsociability, dizziness in the elderly.

Hydrodiuril (hydrochlorothiazide). For edema.

Hydropres (hydrochlorothiazide, reserpine). For high blood pressure.

Hygroton (chlorthalidone). For high blood pressure, edema.

Inderal (propranolol). For angina pectoris, heart rhythm abnormality, pheochromocytoma, high blood pressure.

Indocin (indomethacin). For arthritic conditions.

Ionamin (phentermine resin). For weight reduction.

Isordil (isosorbide dinitrate). For angina pectoris.

Kaon (potassium gluconate). For correcting low blood-potassium levels.

Keflex (cephalexin). For infection.

Kenalog (triamcinolone). For inflammatory skin conditions.

Lanoxin (digoxin). For congestive heart failure, other heart conditions.

Lasix (furosemide). For edema.

Librax (chlordiazepoxide, clidinium bromide). For symptomatic relief of gastrointestinal disturbances.

Librium (chlordiazepoxide). For anxiety, tension.

Lomotil (diphenoxylate, atropine). For diarrhea.

Macrodantin (nitrofurantoin). For urinary tract infection.

Marax (ephedrine sulfate, theophylline, hydroxyzine). For asthma.

Medrol (methylprednisolone). For endocrine and rheumatic disorders, serious skin diseases, allergic states, other conditions.

Mellaril (thioridazine). For psychiatric disorders.

Meprobamate. For anxiety, tension.

Minocin (minocycline). For infection.

Mycolog (nystatin, neomycin, triamcinolone, gramicidin). For some skin conditions.

Mycostatin (nystatin). For fungal infections of mouth, throat.

Mysteclin-F (tetracycline, amphotericin B). For infection.

Nembutal (pentobarbital). For sedation, insomnia.

Neosporin (polymyxin B, neomycin, gramicidin). For skin

infections, infected eczema, herpes, and seborrheic dermatitis.

Nicotinic acid.   For reducing high blood-fat levels.

Nitroglycerin.   For prevention or treatment of anginal attacks.

Noludar (methyprylon).   For insomnia.

Norgesic (orphenadrine, methylbenzhydryl, aspirin, phenacetin, caffeine).   For pain.

Norlestrin (norethindrone, ethinyl estradiol).   Oral contraceptive.

Omnipen (ampicillin).   For infection.

Oracon-21 (ethinyl estradiol, dimethistine).   Oral contraceptive.

Orinase (tolbutamide).   For diabetes.

Ornade (chlorpheniramine, phenylpropanolamine, isopropamide).   For nasal congestion.

Ortho-Novum, Ortho-Novum 1/50-21, Ortho-Novum 1/80-21 (norethindrone, mestranol, in varying dosages).   Oral contraceptive.

Ovral (norgestrel, ethinyl estradiol).   Oral contraceptive.

Ovulen (ethynodiol, mestranol).   Oral contraceptive.

Parafon Forte (chlorzoxazone, acetaminophen).   For acute, painful muscle and skeletal conditions.

Pavabid (papaverine).   For reduced heart and brain blood flow conditions.

Pediamycin (erythromycin).   For infection.

Penbritin (ampicillin).   For infection.

Penicillin G potassium.   For infection.

Penicillin VK (phenoxymethyl penicillin).   For infection.

Pentids (penicillin G potassium).   For infection.

Pen-Vee K (penicillin V potassium).   For infection.

Percodan (oxycodone, aspirin, phenacetin, caffeine).   For pain.

Periactin (cyproheptadine).   For allergies.

Peritrate (pentaerythritol).   For prevention and treatment of angina pectoris.

Phenaphen/codeine (phenacetin, aspirin, phenobarbital, codeine).   For pain and anxiety.

Phenergan (promethazine).   For allergies, motion sickness, nausea/vomiting.

Phenobarbital.   For sedation.

Placidyl (ethchlorvynol).   For insomnia.

Polaramine (dexchlorpheniramine).   For allergy.

Polycillin (ampicillin).   For infection.

Prednisone.   For severe skin and other diseases, hypersensitivity, malignancy.

Premarin (conjugated estrogens).   For amenorrhea, estrogen deficiency states, some abnormal uterine bleeding conditions, prostate cancer.

Principen (ampicillin).   For infection.

Pro-Banthine (propantheline).   For peptic ulcer.

Proloid (thyroglobulin).   For low thyroid function.

Pyridium (phenazopyridine).   For urinary pain, burning, urgency, frequency.

Quinidine sulfate.   For heart rhythm abnormalities.

Rauzide (rauwolfia, bendroflumethiazide).   For high blood pressure.

Regroton (chlorthalidone, reserpine).   For high blood pressure.

Reserpine.   For high blood pressure.

Ritalin (methylphenidate).   For mild depression, some senile behavior states, minimal brain dysfunction in children.

Salutensin (hydroflumethiazide, reserpine).   For high blood pressure.

Ser-Ap-Es (reserpine, hydralazine, hydrochlorothiazide).   For high blood pressure.

Serax (oxazepam).   For anxiety, tension, agitation, irritability.

Sinequan (doxepin).   For anxiety, depression.

Stelazine (trifluoperazine).   For anxiety, tension, agitation, psychotic disorders.

Sterazolidin (phenylbutazone, prednisone, aluminum hydroxide, magnesium trisilicate).   For arthritis, bursitis, gout, acute fibrositis.

Sumycin (tetracycline).   For infection.

Synalar (fluocinolone).   For inflammatory skin conditions.

Talwin (pentazocine).   For moderate to severe pain.

Tandearil (oxyphenbutazone).   For arthritis, gout, painful shoulder, some other inflammatory conditions.

Tedral (theophylline, ephedrine, phenobarbital).   For asthma, bronchitis.

Teldrin (chlorpheniramine maleate). For allergies.
Tenuate (diethylpropion). For weight reduction.
Terramycin (oxytetracycline). For infection.
Tetracycline. For infection.
Tetrex (tetracycline phosphate complex). For infection.
Thorazine (chlorpromazine). For nausea and vomiting, tetanus, agitation, excessive anxiety, tension, psychotic disorders.
Thyroid. For thyroid deficiency.
Tigan (trimethobenzamide). For nausea and vomiting.
Tofranil (imipramine). For depression, childhood bed-wetting.
Tolinase (tolazamide). For diabetes.
Tranxene (chlorazepate). For anxiety.
Triaminic (phenylpropanolamine, pheniramine, pyrilamine). For nasal congestion, postnasal drip.
Triavil (perphenazine, amitriptyline). For anxiety and/or depression.
Tuinal (secobarbital, amobarbital). For insomnia.
Tuss-Ornade (caramiphen, chlorpheniramine, phenylpropanolamine). For cough, upper respiratory congestion, excessive nasal secretion.
Valisone (betamethasone). For inflammatory skin conditions.
Valium (diazepam). For tension, anxiety, muscle spasm.
Vasodilan (isoxsuprine). For blood vessel disorders, threatened abortion.
V-Cillin K (penicillin V potassium). For infection.
Vibramycin (doxycycline). For infection, tourist diarrhea.
Vioform-Hydrocortisone (iodochlorhydroxyquin, hydrocortisone). For some skin disorders.
Vistaril (hydroxyzine). For anxiety, tension, agitation.
Zyloprim (allopurinol). For gout.

Index

DR. HENRY J. HEIMLICH'S reputation extends well beyond the United States. He has lectured in England, France, West Germany, Greece, Israel, Rumania, Japan and throughout South America. Dr. Heimlich is professor of advanced clinical sciences at Xavier University, associate clinical professor of surgery at the University of Cincinnati College of Medicine, and is on the staff of The Deaconess Hospital in Cincinnati.

Educated at Cornell University and Cornell Medical College, Dr. Heimlich served as surgical resident at Mt. Sinai and Bellevue hospitals in New York City. He not only maintains his practice, but finds time as well for teaching and for interviews on national television, radio, and in newspapers. He lectures to medical and other groups around the world on the Heimlich Maneuver, surgery, emergency medicine and "computers for peace." The International Platform Association has designated Dr. Heimlich among the top twenty speakers in the country. He is experimenting in biomedical engineering and continuing research in thoracic surgery and the treatment of cancer. He has just completed work with three other scientists (one of whom is Neil Armstrong, the first man on the moon) on the development of a portable oxygen supply for people who suffer from emphysema and other chronic lung diseases.

LAWRENCE GALTON, perhaps the nation's most respected writer and editor of medical books for the layman, is a former visiting professor at Purdue University. He is a columnist for *Family Circle,* and his articles frequently appear in *The New York Times Magazine, Reader's Digest, Parade,* and other national publications. Writing both his own books and as a collaborator with physicians, he has more than twenty books to his credit.